Praise for *Knocked Up*

"*Knocked Up* is the best cure for morning sickness! *Knocked Up* is the answer to the postpartum blues! *Knocked Up* can cure preeclampsia! Yes, *Knocked Up* can solve gestational diabetes! *Knocked Up* even works on stretch marks! Like Prozac, and safe to take while nursing—this is a hilarious book!"

—Molly Jong-Fast, author of
The Sex Doctors in the Basement and *Normal Girl*

"*Knocked Up* is a delightful story about getting knocked up, popping the baby out, and everything that happens in between. Rebecca Eckler's hilarious and candid account of what seem to be the longest nine months of her life will go down as smoothly as a well-mixed cosmopolitan."

—Amulya Malladi, author of
Serving Crazy with Curry

"Incipient motherhood has never been so sexy. Rebecca Eckler reminds us of something too many people forget—that pregnancy *begins* with an act of lust. She takes us on a wild and funny journey as she stays hip enough and tough enough not to let a simple thing like conception slow her down."

—Claire Scovell LaZebnik, author of
Same as It Never Was

Knocked

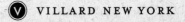

Ⓥ VILLARD NEW YORK

REBECCA ECKLER

Up

Confessions of a Hip Mother-to-be

A Villard Books Trade Paperback

Published in the United States by Villard Books, an imprint of The Random House Publishing Group, a division of Random House, Inc., New York.

VILLARD and "V" CIRCLED Design are registered trademarks of Random House, Inc.

This work was originally published in Canada by Anchor Canada, a division of Random House of Canada Limited, in 2004.

LIBRARY OF CONGRESS CATALOGING-IN-PUBLICATION DATA
Eckler, Rebecca.
Knocked up: confessions of a hip mother-to-be / Rebecca Eckler.
p. cm.
ISBN 0-345-47575-5
1. Eckler, Rebecca. 2. Pregnant women—Biography. 3. Pregnancy—Popular works. 4. Pregnancy—Humor. I. Title: Confessions of a hip mother-to-be. II. Title.
RG525.E335 2005
618.2'0092—dc22
[B]   2004053568

Villard Books website address: www.villard.com

Printed in the United States of America

6 8 9 7 5

For SJC, a.k.a. the fiancé, my favorite person always . . .

And, of course, for Rowan Joely, our baby.

THE FIRST TRIMESTER

a.k.a. The Longest Three Months of My Life

SUNDAY, JANUARY 26

6:45 a.m.
   OH SHIT!

   Did I . . . did we . . . did he . . . in me?

6:46 a.m.

I'm awake, right? I'm conscious, right? I don't feel like myself. Something has changed.

6:47 a.m.

OH MY GOD! The elastic waistband of these boxer shorts can't *already* be tighter. This cannot be happening. To me. Of all people. Oh God . . . I just felt something *moving*.

6:59 a.m.

Oh God, I HAVE THE FEAR!

I can't believe that I . . . that we . . . that he . . . in me.

We did, right?

SHIT!

7:00 a.m.

It's way too early to be so awake on a *Sunday*. I'm going to sneak out of bed and quietly go to the kitchen and reheat what's left of yesterday's midafternoon Starbucks nonfat vanilla latte in the microwave. I need caffeine. There's no way I can fall back to sleep *now*. I need to make the Fear Phone Call *right away*. I desperately need to talk to Lena. But the fiancé is still sleeping, or pretending to still be asleep. How can he possibly be sleeping *at a time like this*? Man, it must be nice to be a man. Men can sleep through anything. It's freaking annoying. I can't let the fiancé know that I'm f-r-e-a-k-i-n-g out. The fiancé can't—under any circumstances—overhear the Fear Conversation I need to have with Lena, as soon as possible. I mean *immediately*. If the fiancé knew what Lena and I really talk about, he would never want anything to do with me—or any other woman—ever again. There is already a good chance that the fiancé already wants nothing to do with me after last night, and I've probably turned him off women forever.

If I were a good person, I would go out and buy the fiancé bagels or something. I am a bad, bad person. Even if the fiancé wasn't here, it's too early to call Lena anyway. When I last remember seeing her, it was two in the morning and she was breakdancing on the dance floor, thrusting her pelvis up toward the ceiling. She didn't look bad either, considering she was a thirty-eight-year-old drunken white girl dancing to Eminem. She, too, will have The Fear this morning and will be sleeping off her hangover until at least noon. Which is what I'd be doing too if The Fear wasn't so devastating and hadn't woken me up like a slap in the face so freaking early. I think I'm hyperventilating.

Did I . . . did we . . . did he . . . in me?
  Shit, shit, shit . . .

The Fear is what happens when vague memories of drunken stupidity instantly become clear as crystal. The only thing to do when the sheer terror of The Fear hits is to go back to bed, bury your head under the comforter, and never, ever leave your house again. Either that or make the Fear Call to your closest girlfriend to try to piece together the puzzle of fogginess by detailing what little you both can remember from the previous night. You can really only stay in bed for so long, no matter how mortified you are.

The Fear Phone Call, the morning after a night of way too much drinking, can last hours. The Fear Phone Call always, always begins with "Oh God, I have *The Fear*" and carries on with much laughter, gossip, and good-natured (and a lot of not-so-good-natured) bitchiness. It always ends with promises to "*never, ever* drink *that* much again."

If this was a typical morning after with The Fear and the fiancé wasn't asleep—or pretending to still be asleep—in the next room, I would tell Lena how I flirted with my boss, that one of my married colleagues came up behind me, wrapped his arms around my waist, and whispered in my ear, "Just because you're engaged now doesn't mean we can't get together, right?" I would tell Lena how I think I remember yelling at a drunken, sloppy guest for spilling her entire drink down the back of my $900 dress so that the material clung to my skin, like a bad date you're trying to lose in a crowd. Or was that me who spilled my drink? In any case, all of that *did* happen at the party last night. But all of that seems kind of innocuous, considering what happened *after* the fiancé and I somehow managed to make it back to my apartment. How did we get back?

Did I . . . did we . . . did he . . . in me?

Lena would tell me how she kissed a man whose name she never knew, and that she doesn't remember how or what time she got home—which is always what happens when Lena drinks too much. We'd laugh until we wept, and we'd groan about our foolishness until our stomachs hurt. We'd reassure each other that what happened in our intoxicated state wasn't so bad. Surely everyone else was too drunk to even notice our bad behavior. Truth is, I look forward to the Fear Phone Call. Actually, I adore the Fear Phone Call. Because if you've made the Fear Phone Call, it usually means you've had an incredible night. The longer the Fear Phone Call lasts, the better and more memorable the night.

But this is not a typical morning with The Fear. I have super freakin' crazy fear. I got into bed last night drunk on alcohol and high on exhilaration, snuggling in with my drunken fiancé, thinking how wonderful my life will be with this man, how much I love him, and how lucky I am that he loves me. I didn't even brush my teeth before pulling him down on top of me. Now I'm anxious and guilt-ridden and sober as a nun. There's a good chance the fiancé will dump me after what happened, after what I *begged him* to do. It was entirely my fault. Sort of.

The fiancé and I celebrated our engagement last night at a party we threw for 150 of our closest friends. The party was also my fault. Everything that happens in a relationship can be blamed on someone, after all. It was my "brilliant idea" to celebrate our engagement. What was I thinking?

I was the one who called him at work one morning, two months ago. "We are having an engagement party. This is what people do when they get engaged. We've been engaged for two months already and I want to celebrate with our friends. We are having a party and I don't care what you say," I informed him. We had fights about the party. He wanted to wait until we were both a little less busy, which would have been never. I told him that he wouldn't have to do a thing, that he'd just have to show up. He wouldn't even have to buy a new outfit. I really meant it, at the time. I did. But then, after I hired the party planner and made my guest list (sixty people I liked, sixty people I didn't, and thirty payback invites), I got bored with it all. The fiancé ended up talking to the party planner more often than I did. He picked the menu (mashed-potato bar, seared ostrich, individual cups of green tea ice cream), the drinks (twelve-year-old scotch and champagne were a must), and the music (top 40 and soul funk). He paid for the whole thing, too (about a year's rent). All of which is typical. It's always me who has the "brilliant" ideas, and then, much to his annoyance, he is invariably left to see them through. The fiancé is responsible and finishes what he sets out to do. I am not responsible and can't even finish a sandwich without getting bored of what I'm eating halfway through. A new rule was created in our relationship as a result of planning our engagement party. "Beck, whenever you have one of your brilliant ideas," he advised, "we are going to have a five-day cooling-off period to decide if it's really something we want to do. That's how it's going to be from now on, okay?"

I agreed.

At least for the guests, the party was a success. We showed that we are a fabulous couple who can throw a fabulous party for our fabulous friends. There was a fabulous open bar, and I got into bed last night feeling like a fabulously sexy woman, on top of the world, a woman who can get away with dancing in six-inch stiletto heels, a woman who has married men hitting on her with her fiancé in the same room, a woman who is comfortable flirting with her boss—I can handle married men hitting on me. I can handle flirting with my boss—it makes work that much more interesting. What I can't handle is what's going on *now*. This cannot be happening to *me* of all people.

I woke up pregnant.

1:00 p.m.

Me? Pregnant? It's like a sick joke, an oxymoron. It's so *not* me. "Lena! Thank God! I have THE FEAR," I cry into the phone. Finally, I was alone, and, finally, Lena had picked up. I had been trying to get through to her for the past five minutes, pushing the redial button as furiously as a crack addict who needs a fix from her dealer. I knew that eventually Lena would pick up. You can only ignore a ringing phone for so long.

"Christ. Was that you who kept calling? Okay, what happened? This better be good. I think I'm still drunk," says Lena. Her voice is froglike. She sounds as though she's been run over by a truck.

So I tell her. "I'm pregnant."

"You are not pregnant," replies Lena, sighing and making some dreadful noise with her throat. "You just have The Fear."

I can't believe it. Don't I deserve more of a reaction than a sigh, a clearing of the throat, and a patronizing tone? I got more of a reaction when I told her, during the last Fear Phone Call, that I found out that our friend Shannon's ex-boyfriend, who broke her heart, had recently slept with another one of our mutual friends, unbeknownst to Shannon. In fact, I got more of a reaction from Lena when I told her Scott Foley and Jennifer Garner split up. What I just told her is so much bigger. It's *life altering*.

The fiancé left about half an hour ago to catch his airplane. I think we were being awkward with each other. He could barely look at me.

"I didn't sleep at all," the fiancé said, shoving a rumpled heap of his clothes into his carry-on luggage.

"Really? Why?" I asked, playing dumb—though I was pleased to learn he had only been pretending to sleep. "I thought for sure you would have passed out." He had drunk a lot too—way too much, in fact. For him to do what he did, he must have been really plowed. He is a corporate lawyer who thinks everything through, which is why I admire him. I think nothing through, which up until now I think he always thought was one of my quirky charms. He really should have known better than to listen to me moaning, "Just come in me. I really want to feel you in me." I mean, really. What happened to the five-day cooling-off period? It was his bright idea to have a cooling-off period in the first place.

"I just didn't sleep," he said, grumpily. The Fear apparently hit him even quicker than it hit me. I had passed out after "it" happened. So at least I had a couple of hours of alcohol-induced slumber. I wonder if the fiancé stayed awake worrying all night about what we had done or if he just couldn't sleep for another reason entirely, like that the room was too warm.

I wanted to pretend that what happened didn't really happen, so I didn't even go through the motions of "Oh, don't worry." I figured that if I didn't bring it up, maybe it wouldn't be real.

Some would say that the fiancé and I have a screwed-up relationship. I say we have a "modern" relationship. We have never lived together, have never really discussed—even after we got engaged—living together. We live in different cities and visit each other a couple of times a month, which means we always miss each other, something I can say about almost no other couple I know who live under the same roof. We are happy the way things are. He has his life and I have my life. When you don't live with your partner, especially when you don't live in the same city as your partner, you can act single. Being in a long-distance relationship is like having the best of both worlds. I'm not quite ready to completely give up my single life. It's way too much fun to flirt. Even after I became an engaged woman and got to walk around with a two-carat diamond ring on my finger I would sometimes forget I wasn't single. The fiancé likes his single life, too. To him, the most awful thing in the world would be if we morphed into one of those boring couples that do everything together, including sharing the same e-mail address. Yuck. We have always said we will NEVER become *one of those couples.* I never come down hard on him when he stays out late with friends because I never really know what time he comes home. He can't yell at me for leaving my dishes on the coffee table for days on end because he doesn't have to see it on a daily basis. We have the perfect relationship.

"I am pregnant," I tell Lena, reheating yesterday's Starbucks latte for the fourth time and lighting a cigarette. I can't be expected to quit just like that. Smoking is an addiction. Plus, I've only known I was pregnant for what, five hours now?

"How did this happen?" Lena asks, suddenly (thankfully) sounding more alert. Maybe my news has just shocked her into nonchalance.

"Well, a boy and a girl get together and get naked and the boy puts his—"

"Okay, stop! You know what I mean."

"Can I blame it on the cosmopolitans? Can I blame it on the dress?" I ask. "It was the cosmos and the dress. It was a toxic mix that made me do things I'd never, ever do sober or while I was wearing jeans and a T-shirt. I should've worn jeans and drunk Perrier all night. My life would be totally different this morning."

I had worn a sexy black dress, the type of dress that it is impossible to wear a bra under. I was showing cleavage, something I am not used to doing and, apparently, something the fiancé is not used to seeing. I think he liked it. Maybe even a little too much. I have always been jealous of women who could show their cleavage off comfortably and fearlessly, like my friend Amy, whose breasts often make public appearances. Amy will say things like "I'm bringing the girls out tonight" when you ask what she plans to wear to a cocktail party. When she "brings out the girls," we know we're going to see her two perfectly round globes of flesh. Not only are Amy's breasts talked to at parties by "tit talkers"—the type of men who look at your breasts while speaking with you—her breasts are also talked about after she leaves. And you know what they say: the only thing worse than being talked about is not being talked about. The same thing is true about breasts. Just one night in my life, I wanted my breasts to be talked about. Is that so wrong?

At last count, I had drunk six cosmopolitans and a couple of flutes of champagne. I should have stopped after two glasses of champagne, which is about the time I first began to feel tipsy. Of course, that was about fifteen minutes after arriving at the party. I have always been a cheap drunk. But I couldn't help but drink a lot last night. It was a celebration, after all! The cosmos, with real cranberries floating around in them, went down like Kool-Aid. I like Kool-Aid. Oh God, I am a twenty-nine-year-old woman who likes Kool-Aid—definitely not mother material. I cannot be pregnant. Except for the fact that I know I am.

"It was an amazing dress," agrees Lena. "And those drinks! They were spectacular. I had about twelve of them."

I can't bring myself to tell her the truth—even

though I tell Lena almost everything. That it is my fault that I'm now pregnant, not entirely the fault of the dress or the booze.

"You are not pregnant," Lena sighs once again. "What are the chances?"

"You're right. But I do feel different. I feel pregnant."

"How could you possibly know you're pregnant five hours after having unprotected sex? What exactly are you feeling?"

"Well, for starters, I have a headache and I feel nauseous, like I have morning sickness. I'm queasy, like I could throw up any second."

"Oh my God!" says Lena, enunciating each word. "You have a hangover! Ouch. Don't make me yell at you. My whole body hurts. You have a headache and feel like throwing up? So do I! Maybe I'm pregnant too! Sadly, I didn't have sex last night, but we do share the same symptoms. I'm probably pregnant as well."

"Enough, enough. I see your point. You're right. You're right," I agree. "I just have a hangover. There's no way I could have sex one time without protection and end up pregnant. There's no way. But Lena?"

"Y-e-s-s-s-s?"

"I am pregnant."

"I'm going back to bed. I'll call you later. You are not pregnant. I have The Fear too. Do you know that I can't remember how I got home? I think I remember kissing someone in a taxi and jumping out before it went further. I'm not sure who the guy was, though. I am *never, ever* drinking *that* much again."

That's Lena. Though I have just shared the biggest news, taking the Fear Phone Call to a new level, the conversation always comes back to her. It's sort of her charm. You learn to love it after a while.

"Lena, do you know that while you were break-dancing to Eminem, a child was conceived?" I tell her.

I can out-self-obsess her. That's my charm.

"You could name the child Cosmo," says Lena. "You know, after the drinks."

The Fear Call ends abruptly. I hang up on Lena.

JANUARY 27

I couldn't sleep at all last night. I took three Advils to try to scare off the headache, which lasted all day. I am not ecstatic to maybe be pregnant. The fiancé and I haven't even discussed a wedding date yet. We haven't even discussed when the next time we are going to *see* each other will be. Before he got on his plane yesterday, the fiancé didn't call me from the airport like he usually does. Which is a good thing. I'm sure if he had called to tell me he loves me before he got on his plane, like he usually does, I would have said something stupid like "I think I may be pregnant," and, with those six words, I would have ruined not only his plane ride, but his life. I can hold off ruining his life. At least for a couple more days.

Being pregnant is definitely going to ruin my life, a life which was pretty simple but thoroughly enjoyable. My life is about partying with friends, Fear Phone Calls the morning after, going to spin classes so my ass can fit into low-rise jeans, and writing columns for a newspaper. I get paid a good salary and I work only a couple of hours a day, spending the rest of my time talking on the phone with friends. Twice a month I visit the fiancé. The maximum reward for the minimum effort was all working out just fine by me.

I'm quite sure the fiancé and I would not get along as well if we lived together under the same roof. Saturday morning, for example, he got into a funk after I left a wet towel on the bed, again. "It's like I have a child as a partner," he said, storming out of the bedroom. He uses that line on me a lot. "It's like I have a child for a partner," he will say when we go out to eat and I order chicken fingers off the children's menu. I like chicken fingers. "It's like I have a child," he will say when he sees me making ice cream sandwiches with waffles. I like waffle ice cream sandwiches. "It's like I have a child for a partner," he will say when I leave the cap off the toothpaste, which, really, I don't think is the biggest deal. How guilty do I really need to feel leaving a gob of Colgate on the sink counter? It's not like I'm an inside trader or a murderer.

If I am *not* pregnant, I will never, ever again leave a wet towel on the bed. At least, if I am *not* pregnant, I will never, ever again leave a wet towel on *his* side of the bed. At the very least, if I am *not* pregnant, I will never, ever again leave a wet towel on his side of the bed when he's visiting. I'm pretty sure I can live up to that, if I'm *not* pregnant.

The fiancé is kind of right, though. I am twenty-nine years old and not mother material. What kind of mother prefers Froot Loops to Special K for breakfast? What kind of mother gets her home phone cut off four times a year because she forgets to pay her bill? What kind of mother owns only three forks, one knife, two spoons, and twelve free promotional mugs that were sent to her at work? I don't even own oven mitts. The one time I needed to pick up a hot plate in the kitchen, I used my bath mat. I forget to water my plants for months. I don't even know how the plants got into my apartment in the first place. I know I have never actually purchased any plants, so their presence in my living room is a complete mystery.

The worst thing about being pregnant right now would be that I was so very close to reaching my goal of having Janet Jackson abs. Thanks to hours a week at the gym and a regular personal trainer, my stomach has never been flatter than it is right now. My career, writing the Girl Column for the newspaper, has just started to take off as well. My entire raison d'être relies on my living a fabulous life, going to trendy bar openings and parties, so I can gather material to write about being a young woman in the city. Even if I'm not always having the best time, it's my job to make it seem like I am always having a better time than everyone else. If I get fat, some skinny, younger girl reporter with a stomach as flat as a countertop will get my job and do it better, and I will be fired. This whole thing is a disaster.

How could I have been so stupid? I have ruined my life. I am never having sex again. I mean, I am never having unprotected sex again. Unprotected sex, like that black dress I wore the other night, is a bad idea. Ten minutes of great sex and my life is over. But another life has just begun. Life apparently does not happen when you're busy making other plans. Life is what happens when there is an open bar.

JANUARY 28

10:00 a.m.

Maybe I haven't completely ruined my life. Isn't it better to be a young mother, like Reese Witherspoon, than an old mother, like Madonna? Reese has managed to have two kids before the age of twenty-eight. She always looks stunning on red carpets and makes $15 million a picture. She's America's Sweetheart! Because I am young(ish), my body will bounce back quicker if I have a baby now. My eggs won't be healthy forever. Lena, who is thirty-eight and still single, is always moaning about how her eggs are old and her ovaries have probably dried up like prunes. I did want kids eventually, didn't I? This way, my child will be in school full-time, and I'll only be thirty-five. Some people don't even decide what they want to do with their lives until they're thirty-five. Right now is actually the most perfect time to be pregnant. I'm employed. My newspaper has benefits. I can take maternity leave. I can still work from home after giving birth. The fiancé will be a great father.

The fiancé is actually ideal father material. I've said this many times. "He's definitely marriage and father material," I would say to my friends when the fiancé and I first started dating, and they would nod, knowing exactly what I meant. Women always know what "father material" means when you describe a man you're dating that way. It means that the guy is a perfect mix of provider and protector, brains and brawn, that he always takes your phone calls no matter how busy he is at work.

Sure, this pregnancy is unplanned. But some of the best things in my life have been unplanned. I didn't plan to be a newspaper reporter. I didn't plan to fall in love and be in a long-distance relationship for five years. Shit happens. And, for the most part, all the unplanned things in my life have worked out just fine. It's like when you plan just to go out for brunch and then spontaneously decide to go shopping and end up finding the one pair of pants that makes your ass look like a ripe peach. It's actually a good thing.

10:20 a.m.

Who am I kidding? The fiancé will dump me. My boss will fire me. My parents will never talk to me again. I will be a single, unemployed, unwed mother who keeps in touch with the father of her child only through support checks. I have ruined my life and that of this unborn child.

JANUARY 29

No one believes me. My other best friend, Ronnie, refuses to acknowledge that there's even the slightest possibility that I'm knocked up. It's not like I utter the words "I'm pregnant!" every day. I'm kind of hurt no one is taking me seriously.

"You are not pregnant," Ronnie told me, laughing into the phone. I had assumed Ronnie would understand what I'm going through. We are the same age but live entirely different lives. She has three children, all under the age of five. We attended college together. She got married right after graduation, while I took on a very important job serving coffee to guests in the waiting room of a nightly television current affairs talk show. At the time I was sleeping with a drummer in a band the name of which is too painful to repeat. Ronnie was nearly a virgin when she got married. (She had slept with only two men, and one of those two men she only half-screwed. To this day, she's not even sure what happened.) She had her first child at

21

twenty-five, her second at twenty-seven, and her third at twenty-nine. We speak almost every day—for about three minutes. Without fail, her kids start screaming in the background and she must rush off to attend to them, because this is what mothers do. And Ronnie is a very good mother. While she's driving her kids to daycare or school or music lessons, I'm usually still sleeping. While she's busy baking cookies for fundraisers that will guarantee that her children get into good private schools, I'm partying with friends. I know her kids' names but for the life of me I couldn't tell you their birthdays. I practically yelled at her four-year-old son when I called her this morning.

"Brad? I need to speak to your mommy," I said.

"My mommy?"

"Yes, your mommy. Is she there?"

"Yeth."

"Can I speak to her? Please?"

"Yeth."

"Um, Brad sweetie? Get your mommy NOW!"

"Who ith this?" My God, is my kid going to be this stupid? Of course, Brad is four. Maybe all four-year-olds are stupid.

"It's your mommy's friend Rebecca. Where is your mommy?"

"I don't know. Do you like Harold?"

"No. I don't like Harold. Who is Harold?" Argh. Why did I take the bait?

"He's Ms. Thompson's bird." Not going to ask who Ms. Thompson is. Not going to ask.

"Brad. I really, really need to speak to your mother. *Please* tell her to come to the phone."

"My daddy drives a car."

"Yes, your daddy is very smart. Where. Is. Your. Mother?"

"I have a penith. My mommy hath a vagina." How the hell do you respond to that?

"Please, Brad. Your mommy will give you chocolate cake if you go get her for me *right now*."

"Who ith this?" I'm going to snap. I am.

"It's your mommy's friend. Get her NOW."

"She doethn't like you."

"Yes she does."

"You are not nice."

"Yes I am."

"Do you drive a car like my daddy?"

I know it was wrong to get infuriated with the kid. But he's not my kid. And, yeth, I really needed to thpeak to his mommy. What does he not understand about "Get your mommy NOW"?

Then, suddenly, Brad put the phone down. What followed was about a minute and a half of silence on the other end.

"Hello?" said Ronnie, finally picking up the phone. "Is someone there?"

"Thank God!" I huffed, exasperated.

"Hey, did you just call me? I didn't even hear it ring."

Jesus. This is why kids should never be allowed to pick up a phone. Ever.

"I know I am pregnant," I told Ronnie, once

again, before explaining what happened the night of the engagement party. "I know my body. I know something is different. Stop laughing!"

"I'm sorry. I'm sorry. Were you ovulating?"

"Why? Does that matter? How the hell do I know if I was ovulating? What does ovulation have to do with getting pregnant?"

"Um, everything? I thought you knew your body. Some women can feel when they're ovulating. When was your last period?"

"I'm not sure. I think it was . . . I don't know."

What type of woman actually keeps track of her periods anyway? The type that has a lot of sex, I suppose. And the type that is super organized and owns Filofaxes or Palm Pilots so she can write that sort of thing down and fill up her calendar so it looks like she lives a very busy, very organized life. I am neither of these types. Before I would have even protected sex with a man, I would make him run down his sexual history with me. I would ask, "When was the last time you had an AIDS test?" Much to his horror, I made my fiancé actually take an AIDS test before I would sleep with him. Men will do almost anything if they want to sleep with you, even if it means taking the morning off work and spending four hours in a public health clinic. The last time I wrote something down in my Filofax was in 1998, in one of my "brilliant idea" flashes, when I decided it would be a "brilliant idea" to get organized. During those four days of organization, I never once even thought about writing down "Period today."

"Beck, I'm sorry. I've got to run. I have a kid screaming in each room and I have to make dinner. I'll have to call you tomorrow, Mama," Ronnie said, before we even made it to the three-minute mark.

"Oh God. Don't say that to me! Do not say that to me!" I think I actually felt my heart skip a beat at being called "Mama." It was like when I'm forced to listen to jazz. I hate the sound of it.

"I'm joking. Find out when your last period was, okay? You are not pregnant. You are just being psycho, girl. Once you find out when your last period was, you can figure out if you were ovulating or not. You can log on to the Internet and type in 'ovulation calculator' and type in the date of your last period, and it will tell you if you were fertile the night of your engagement party. That's what I did when I was trying to get pregnant with Brad."

"Okay, okay. Wow. I didn't even know about that. Listen, one more quick question and then I'll let you go. Did you feel morning sickness the day after you got pregnant?"

"I'm definitely getting off the phone now. And no, I did not. You cannot possibly have morning sickness two days after you've conceived. It doesn't hit for four to six weeks."

"But, I swear, I think I can feel the baby *moving*."

"But it's not even a baby yet! It's like nothing. It's like a spot! In a few weeks, when you get your period, you'll be laughing too. We'll be laughing about this over a bottle of wine. Trust me. You're just being a drama queen."

Actually, we will not be laughing about this or anything else over a bottle of wine. Ever since Ronnie had children, I can't remember her ever drinking more than one glass of wine. And I still don't see how me being pregnant is so funny. And, for the record, I think that getting pregnant without thinking about it, while the father of the child lives in a different city, is a good reason to be a drama queen.

I don't understand why no one will believe me. I knew practically the minute the fiancé rolled off of me that I was pregnant. It's like how I always know when the phone company is about to cut off my phone. Or how I know, halfway through drying my hair, if I'm going to have a good or bad hair day. It's women's intuition.

JANUARY 30

Ever since the fiancé left, he's been acting weird. Because the fiancé is being weird with me, he's making me be weird with him, and so our dozen or so daily conversations are entirely weird. Ever since *that night,* it's like we have a big weird cloud over our relationship.

"You're being weird," I started our most recent phone call, which started almost exactly like the phone call before that, and the one before that, and the one before that, and the one before that.

"I'm not being weird," he responded. "You're being weird."

"I'm not being weird. I know that you're being weird, though."

"You're the one being weird."

If we both didn't have jobs to attend to, it's possible we could have gone on like that for hours.

"I'm not being weird. I'm being tired," he finally said.

"Me too. I'm being tired. Let's talk later," I said, before throwing in "Weirdo" and hanging up. I always get the last word.

And that's pretty much how we've been talking to each other these days.

Thanks to my favorite shopping buddy, Dana, I have nearly figured out when my last period was.

"Why are you calling me so late in the middle of the week, asking me when you got your last period?" she said groggily when she picked up her phone. "Why are you being so weird?"

Really, is it so weird to call a friend after midnight to ask when you got your last period?

"I am not being weird. I just really, really want to know when we went shopping for those Miu Miu slingbacks. What day was that? Please help me. I need to know."

"Okay, okay. Chill out. What is your problem? You bought those shoes on January 14th. Don't you remember me saying how I couldn't believe John ditched me a month before Valentine's Day, then I spent hundreds of dollars I don't have on clothes I don't need to kill the depression? And don't you remember how I got mad at you for buying those shoes because I really, really wanted them? And then we went to buy you tampons."

"Right, right. Perfect."

"Why? Hey, are you planning to take the shoes back? It's probably too late. But I might be convinced to buy them from you. Can you believe that idiot ditched me a month before Valentine's Day after I spent so long with him? I really trained that guy. He was almost ready to be husband material."

"No, I'm not giving the shoes to you. And, no, I can't believe he dumped you. But, really, you weren't even sure what the guy did for a living, were you? I don't think he was actually marriage material. You should know how your husband spends his days. But I can't talk about that right now. Go back to bed. I'll call you later."

"By the way—great party last weekend. It was the best party I've ever been to. Your dress was amazing. Didn't I tell you you should wear that dress? You looked fantastic. I was right. You should always listen to me."

"Dana, I hate that dress. I'm pregnant."

"WHAT?!?" screeched Dana. Finally, the reaction I was expecting. "When did that happen? You were drinking like a wino at your party."

"No, it happened *the night of* the party. He . . .
you know . . . in me. We were drunk!"

"Are you a fucking idiot?"

"Dana, you must learn to express your opinions. Why don't you tell me how you're really feeling about my accident? We were drunk! And, yes,
I'm a complete fucking idiot."

"Okay, don't freak out. I've been through this
before a couple of times. I always worried that I was
pregnant immediately after too. Chances are
you're not. Okay, that was how many days ago?
Five? Hmm. Too late for a morning-after pill.
I've done that twice. It's easy. You just have to call
your doctor."

"You have?" I couldn't hide my shock. Dana,
in addition to being my favorite shopping buddy,
is also my calorie-counter friend. She's always
counting calories and can tell you exactly how
many calories are in the top of a bran muffin or a
cup of frozen yogurt or a bowl of cereal. It's quite
an amazing skill she has, if a completely odd and
obsessive one. Dana works at a magazine, in the
marketing department, and has the best wardrobe
of all of my friends. I know exactly how many pairs
of shoes she has (fifty-six) but had no idea she had
all that much sex.

"Yeah, well, it's a little late for any sort of
morning-after pill. Not that I'm sure I would be
comfortable doing that anyway. I am turning
thirty soon," I reminded her. "It's not like I'm
sixteen or anything."

"So you want to be pregnant?"

"No, I'm not saying that. I'm just saying . . . okay, I don't know what I'm saying. But don't you think the chances are very, very, very slim that I am?"

"I don't know. Sure."

"Come on. At least pretend with me that it's a long shot. No pun intended."

"Okay. You are not pregnant," said Dana, in a monotone. "But you know, I'm not sure how comfortable those slingbacks will be when your ankles start to swell. Maybe you should give them to me in case you *are* pregnant."

"You are not—under any circumstances—getting those shoes," I told her. "Even if my ankles do swell. Does that happen?"

"Uh, yeah."

"Well, there's $350 down the drain."

"Yeah, and just wait to see what pregnancy does to your ass."

JANUARY 31

Being pregnant is already totally ruining my life. I stayed in tonight—a Friday night—to play Ovulation Calculator on the Internet. I realized instantly that ovulation calculators are addictive. They're like crack. Not that I've ever done crack, but I've never done an ovulation calculator either. I can't get enough of them. Once I remembered shoe shopping with Dana and then going to the drugstore to buy tampons, I felt I was well on my way to figuring out if I was ovulating the night of the party.

Type "ovulation calculator" into any search engine on the Internet and a number of sites pop up on your computer screen. They all ask you to enter the First Day of your Last Period (FDLP) and ask how long your cycle is, and then, poof, your most fertile days of the month will pop up within three seconds. I typed in January 13, holding my breath.

I do not want to be a drama queen, but, according to the twenty-three ovulation calculators I tried, my most fertile days of the month were January 24 to January 28. The fiancé and I "did it"—or, to be more precise, he "did it" in me—on either January 25 or January 26, depending on whether you consider 3 a.m. the night of one or the morning of the other. In either case, I was, apparently, at my most fertile. Did you know that sperm can live up to seventy-two hours in your body? Meaning that even if we didn't do it exactly when I was ovulating, the sperm could have lived on until I was.

All this raises the question, what were the chances that the fiancé and I would have our engagement party on the exact same night that I was at my most fertile? Was it fate? Is "It's fate!" a good, solid argument to use on your fiancé, who lives in a different city, to convince him that having a child is the right thing to do? My fiancé does not believe in fate, which is why I'm pretty sure the whole "It's fate" argument won't get me very far. I hate arguing with lawyers—it's that much more difficult. I believe in fate, but I also believe in fortune tellers and that everyone in the world should like me. My fiancé is always telling me that I "live in a dream world" and that in "the real world," not everyone has to like me. I always argue back that living in a dream world is better than living in the real world, which, I suppose, is where most consultants, stockbrokers, and lawyers live. Most of my friends—artists, television personalities, and writers—live in the dreamy place I inhabit. The "real world" is for people who pay their bills on time. I'm glad I don't live there, even with creditors after me. Maybe, just maybe, in both our worlds the fiancé's sperm wasn't working that night. In the dream world, there's always hope. Though I am sure I am pregnant.

FEBRUARY 1

I keep picturing this itty-bitty little drunken sperm dancing around in my belly. Is it possible for a sperm to be too drunk to make it up into my egg? Is it possible for a sperm to be too drunk to know what it's doing? I mean, the fiancé and I were certainly too drunk to know what *we* were doing. I keep picturing the sperm dancing around, smoking a butt, partying it up the night of our engagement party, and then waking up the next morning with a hangover, just like us. If people get hangovers, then certainly sperm must. "No, I'm too hungover to do my thing today," the sperm would say to itself. "I'm going to pass out now. This gal will just have to get knocked up some other time." Could that have happened?

I really should have paid attention during those Grade 6 sex education classes. I know nothing—absolutely nothing—about the female reproductive system. Now I'm thinking maybe I should send an anonymous e-mail to the human resources department at my office, suggesting sex education classes for adults instead of the yoga and Weight Watchers classes I'm always getting e-mails about, which take place on the third floor in one of the boardrooms once a week. I had no idea about Most Fertile Times of the Month. I had no idea that the First Day of your Last Period was so important. I just thought periods were a bitch, something women had to go through once a month, giving us the opportunity to start arguments with our boyfriends. I didn't realize periods happened for a *reason*.

I could barely get any work done all week. Knowing something is going on in my body makes it hard to concentrate on writing stories about Why Bangs Are Back, and Internet Dating, and Cooking Classes for Singles.

I have done the ovulation calculator 283 times so far. No matter how many times I play with it—

typing in the 12th, 13th, or 14th of the month—I
was still at my most fertile the night the fiancé and
I had unprotected sex, the night I uncharacteristi-
cally moaned, in the throes of passion, "Come on,
I just want to feel you in me. Just stay in me." It
just figures.

FEBRUARY 3

The fiancé just called me at work, interrupting my
investigative work on the most expensive martini
in town, to ask me a question that caught me completely off guard.

"When was the first day of your last period?" he
asked, after (at least) saying "Hello."

Christ. Does absolutely everyone in the world
know about the FDLP?

"What? I'm sorry. What did you just ask me?
Please tell me you didn't ask me what I think you
just asked me." My fiancé and I do not have this
type of relationship. We have a closed-door type
of relationship. Meaning we do not walk around
naked in front of each other. If I'm feeling really
wild, I'll have sex with the lights on, but always
under the sheets. I do not tell the fiancé about my
waxing appointments. It's too personal. It's better, I think, that he just assumes I come all hair-
less and smooth. In the five years we've been
dating, I have never gone to the washroom in
front of him and he has never gone to the wash-

room in front of me. I do not even like him watching me blow-dry my hair. I want him to think I come *perfect*. For his part, he even shuts the door when he clips his toenails. Which is why I love him. I would like our relationship to remain somewhat mysterious. Which is why I don't really want to discuss my period with him. *Ever.* But if we must, shouldn't we really start off by talking about something a little less private, like what kind of deodorant I use, then work our way up to period talk?

"I said, when was your last period?" the fiancé asked again.

"I'm not sure," I responded. I didn't want him to know that I did know, all too well. I wanted to play it breezy. It wouldn't sound so breezy if I answered, immediately, "Around January 14th," as if it were the only thing on my mind. Which it is. But I didn't want him to know that.

"What do you mean, you're not sure? Don't you keep track of these things?" The fiancé was not, apparently, even attempting to be breezy for my sake. He sounded kind of jumpy. He had sounded less panicky, in fact, when he had asked me to *marry* him.

How was I going to answer this potential land mine of a question?

"Well, babe. When was the last time I cried uncontrollably about nothing? Do you remember? Because that's probably when I got my period last," I said.

"You do that once a week," he huffed. So he does pay attention. Good boy.

"Do not," I responded.

"Do too," he responded.

"Well, do you remember the date you first told me you loved me?" I asked him.

"Not now, Beck. I'm not in the mood," he sighed into the phone.

I will not get into a fight with the fiancé over my period. But, for the record, I do think that remembering when you first told the woman you are spending the rest of your life with that you love her is way more important than remembering when the First Day of your Last Period was. Periods happen once a month. Falling in love, if you're lucky, happens but a few times in your *entire* life.

"Okay, fine," I told him. "I think it was around the 13th or 14th."

"Thank you! Was that so hard?" he asked.

"Why do you want to know so badly, anyway?"

"Oh, no reason. Just curious. I'm going to book you a ticket to come see me soon. I'll call you tonight. I have to get back to work."

Shit. The fiancé knows about the ovulation calculators. Why else would he be so hell-bent on knowing when the First Day of my Last Period was? I bet that right now he's typing the date into his computer. Fuck. How is it possible that he knows about ovulation calculators? What kind of man knows about that? I'm going to kill whoever told him about them. I really, truly am.

It is almost impossible to get pregnant. It's amazing any woman gets pregnant at all. It *is* a miracle. Normal fertile couples, I learned doing "research"—it's amazing how much one can learn spending hours typing "early pregnancy symptoms" and "how to get pregnant" into search engines—have only a 25 percent chance of getting pregnant each month. There are dozens and dozens, if not hundreds, of chat rooms for women who experience fertility problems. Most doctors don't even consider looking into possible fertility problems until a year of trying to get pregnant has gone by unsuccessfully. So if I am pregnant, I must be the most fertile woman in the world. Or the fiancé must have supersperm. I had no idea that 14 million sperm are released with every ejaculation. And only a couple hundred survive from that, and then only one has to penetrate the egg. What are the chances that one itty-bitty sperm, one 1,000th of an inch long, managed to strike my egg at just the right angle, at just the right time? Make that, what are the chances that one itty-bitty *drunk* sperm, one 1,000th of an inch long, managed to strike my *drunk* egg at just the right angle, at just the right time? I could barely walk upright when we got home that night. How could the sperm possibly manage to swim straight? I could, if I'm pregnant, be a poster child for a condom manufacturer. My face could be plastered on bus shelter advertisements for birth control pills. I could go around visiting high school students, telling them the importance of protection. One time? Nah, the chances I'm pregnant are next to nil. I can't even get my VCR to work and I've had it for ten years. How is it possible that in ten minutes, without actually knowing how anything in my body works, I could be pregnant? It makes no sense.

FEBRUARY 5

SPERM STUFF I MUST SOMEHOW WORK INTO CONVERSATION WITH THE FIANCÉ

1. "Hey, we should go out for dinner at that new steak restaurant everyone is talking about. Do you know that in some cultures, people eat bulls' testicles? Speaking of which, we've never talked about your testicles. Anything you want to tell me? Are they in good working order?"

2. "Have you noticed that super-tight jeans are coming back in style? I just read that in *Vogue.* Have you ever worn super-tight jeans? Ever?"

3. "We're both pretty stressed out. Maybe we should go away for a spa weekend somewhere nice. Have you been to a spa lately? Have you visited any hot tubs, saunas, or whirlpools lately?"

4. "Can you please pass me the salt? Say, how many cups of coffee do you drink a day?"
5. "So how's that working out coming along? What exactly do you do at the gym? More specifically, how often do you ride a bike?"

This is all so I can figure out if the fiancé's sperm are healthy. I have never seen him in super-tight jeans, which I've always really appreciated, up until right about now. Because he hasn't ever worn tight jeans, he's also to blame for being so damn fertile. Right?

There are also things women can do to increase their fertility. For example, relaxing. Luckily, I'm bad at relaxing. Relaxation—or the attempt at relaxation—stresses me out. Some of the websites suggest that I get to know my basal body temperature. I don't know what basal body temperature is, nor do I own a thermometer. I always thought that basal was an herb.

FEBRUARY 6

8:30 p.m.

I need a pack of cigarettes. I need a gallon of wine to go with my pack of cigarettes. So I'm heading to Triumph, a trendy local haunt, to meet Heather and Shannon, two of my closest friends, whom I haven't seen since the night of my engagement party, a.k.a. the night I got pregnant.

The nausea I was experiencing for a week after my engagement party—the nausea that I thought was morning sickness—has subsided, so maybe it was just a very brutal hangover. I will not tell Heather and Shannon anything, though I kind of want to—for shock value.

We all work in the incestuous industry known as The Media. Heather works as a publicist and has recently ventured out into the world of party planning. She has an on-again-off-again boyfriend. Shannon hosts her own design show on one of those obscure digital cable channels you wonder who watches. She does not have a boyfriend. Shannon and Heather are my "fun" friends. Often when I'm around them, I feel like I'm back in high school, hanging with the cool kids. They are always dressed head to toe in designer clothing, and they always know the hip places to go and the right drinks to order. The three of us always stay out late. Because we work in the same industry, which, like any industry, is a very small world, news of my pregnancy woes would get around too fast. Of course, Heather and Shannon would promise me they would never breathe a word to anyone, but I know they would go straight home and call other people to tell them, making those people "promise" not to tell anyone. And, of course, those people would "promise" and then tell other people.

I also worry that if I tell them, I'll be ousted from the little "club" we have formed. Pregnant women are not so fabulous, after all. They can't drink. They can't smoke. They can't stay out late hitting on men to get free drinks. Shannon has had a few long-time boyfriends. Her relationships have always ended because Shannon makes no secret that she is thirty-three years old and wants to get married and make babies. Unfortunately for her, the guys she is always attracted to do not want to get married and make babies. They'd rather be DJs and have threesomes with wannabe models. Heather, with the on-again-off-again boyfriend, always wants what she doesn't have. When her relationship is "on," she wonders if it would be better to be single. When her relationship isn't working out and she's single, she always wants a boyfriend. I'm the balancing friend. Being in a long-distance relationship, I'm useful when they need a single friend around to go out and meet men with. I'm also useful when they want the perspective or advice of someone in a serious relationship. No, it's better not to tell them anything. It's best to pretend nothing is going on in my life at all.

Midnight

I left Shannon and Heather at the bar. They were still going strong. I managed to get out, having had one glass of wine and a couple of cigarettes. After all, I figure, I don't know anything for sure and I don't want them to think anything is out of the ordinary. While I was around Heather and Shannon, I managed to almost forget about maybe being pregnant. We talked about what we always talk about when we get together: relationships, boys, relationships, and boys. Do women ever talk about anything else? They both kept asking me when I thought I would be getting married. "Come on!" said Heather. "I've never been a bridesmaid before. I want to be a bridesmaid. You have to get married so I can be a bridesmaid."

"Are you kidding? I can't even think about a wedding now. That engagement party took everything out of me. It feels like I have already planned a wedding," I told them.

Professing a headache, I left. They were both on their fourth glass of wine. In the taxi home, I thought about the conversation I had had with Ronnie earlier in the day, when I had broken the news that I had been at my most fertile the night the fiancé . . . in me.

"You have to do a home pregnancy test," Ronnie told me. In just over a week I will be able to do this. It's amazing that they can put a man on the moon and put phones on airplanes and package sliced meat so it stays fresh for weeks, but no genius scientist out there can come up with a home pregnancy test you can do immediately after you've had unprotected sex. I know—I've done the research.

I really did almost feel back to my old self tonight, until I was getting ready for bed and saw something peeking out from under it. It was The Dress: I had forgotten about it after my drunken romp in the sack. I, of course, did what any woman would do when spotting The Dress that had possibly ruined her life. I kicked it farther underneath the bed, where it could be forgotten about for a long while longer. Like I said, I'm never wearing The Dress again anyway. Ever. It's a dangerous, dangerous dress.

FEBRUARY 7

At least the fiancé and I have started to have more normal, longer-than-three-minute conversations once again. He's booked me a ticket to come see him in one week, on Valentine's Day. I'm very much looking forward to the visit. I miss him. I feel like we have to have sex to save our relation-ship—ironic, since sex is what has possibly ruined our relationship in the first place. I think it's a good sign that he wants to see me on Valentine's Day. You can't ditch a girl on Valentine's Day, can you?

I went out with Lena tonight, to a bar where the men wear tight black ribbed turtlenecks and the girls wear tank tops and open-toe heels even though it's the middle of winter and there's a foot of snow on the ground. I was wearing tight jeans, which still fit. I indulged in a glass of red wine and a couple of smokes. I'm going to pretend I live in France, where this is acceptable behavior for a pregnant woman. Now is not the time to quit. I don't need more stress in my life.

"Oh, don't worry. You're not pregnant," said Lena again, refusing to indulge me.

"I'm not sure I should be drinking this," I told her, as the waitress placed our drinks on the table.

"Oh, don't worry about that. All of our mothers drank and smoked like sailors when they were pregnant. Why do you think they didn't gain that much weight? And. You. Are. Not. Pregnant. How many times do I have to tell you that?"

"But I think I have all the symptoms," I told her. "I've spent hours researching early pregnancy symptoms and I have them all! Except the missed period part. I'll have to wait another week to find that out. Lena, are you listening to me?"

Lena was busy eyeing the door to see if anyone she knew had come in and if there were any possible conquests to be had, while giving the other women in the bar the once-over, to size up her competition.

"Yeah, yeah. I'm listening. You have symptoms. What are they?"

"I'm moody. *Very* moody. And I'm so tired all the time. And I'm emotional. This woman on the street today almost made me cry when she walked into me by accident. I had this urge to slap her, and then tears sprang to my eyes. What's that about? And I feel kind of queasy when I wake up."

"Don't take this the wrong way, Beck," said Lena, "but you are always moody. You are always emotional. You are always tired. You are queasy because you are making yourself sick with worry. It would be very hard to tell by those symptoms if you really are pregnant or if you are just being your good ol' bitchy self."

"I'm going to pretend you didn't say that. I think my breasts are bigger. Do they look bigger to you?"

"I don't think so."

"I'm going to visit the fiancé in a week. I'll get him to check my boobs."

"Does he know you're freaking out about this?"

"I think he's freaking, too. I think he knows I know he's freaking like I know he knows I'm freaking. But we pretend we don't know."

"Don't even worry about it until you can take a test. Hey, where's the waiter? I need another drink. Check out that guy over there. He's kind of cute, right? But I'm not sure about his pants. They're a little too suburban or something. Should I go meet him, or what?"

"Just use a condom if you do," I suggested to her. "That's my only advice. Use a condom."

I suppose this is why women pay for therapy. Sometimes friends just don't listen long enough.

FEBRUARY 8

The thing about maybe, possibly being pregnant is that you can't get it out of your mind that you maybe, possibly are pregnant. No matter how much you want to forget about it, you can't. All you are left to do is to think of things like the type of pregnant woman you would like to be and the type you definitely don't want to be.

If I am pregnant, I would like to be as sexy as that infamous photo of a very pregnant Demi Moore on the cover of *Vanity Fair,* or like the very pregnant Brooke Shields, proudly flaunting her belly on the cover of *Vogue.* It would be great to be like the very pregnant Academy Award winner Catherine Zeta-Jones, who attended the Oscars even though she looked like she was about to go into labor at any second. I would like to be the type of pregnant woman who loses all her weight three seconds after giving birth, like Sarah Jessica Parker and Elizabeth Hurley and Kate Moss and every other woman who gives birth in Hollywood or New York. I would also like to be like Jennifer Aniston's character on *Friends,* who had the most amazing maternity wardrobe.

I know the type of pregnant woman I definitely do not want to be. I do not want to be the type who bores all my friends by always talking about how I'm feeling and what I'm going through (though it may *already* be too late for that). I do not want to turn into an overanxious, health-freak hypochondriac who won't leave her house for fear of inhaling car fumes. I definitely do not want to become the type of pregnant woman who, because it's easier, decides to cut her hair above her ears. I do not want to become boring and wear 1980s-style stretchy pants. And I absolutely do not want to join a mommies' group. I'm not even sure I like other mommies that much.

I'm not sure why I'm so consumed by all of this. Like all the friends I've told have said, what are the chances?

It's really the fiancé's parents' fault that I might be pregnant. Not that I'm pointing fingers. Our engagement party was originally scheduled for the 18th, but they had a wedding to attend that night. We moved the party back one week, to the 25th. When you think about it—as I have—if they hadn't had that wedding to go to, everything would have turned out so very differently. One week earlier, I wouldn't have been at my most fertile time. Still, his parents didn't force me, in my drunken state, to beg their son to stay inside of me. But I beg their son to do a lot of things for me and he doesn't listen. Why did he listen that night? So it's his fault too.

Women have an inherent skill, which men don't have, for twisting and changing reality to meet their needs. I once attended a dinner party with six married couples. I posed the question to the men, "How many of you guys proposed only after your wife told you that you had to?" Five of the six couples admitted it was the woman who first brought up that she wanted to get married. You never hear engaged or married women saying, "Oh, it was so romantic. I begged and pleaded and threatened to walk out on him until he proposed." You only ever hear, "Oh, it was so romantic. He got down on one knee and told me how he couldn't imagine his life without me, and then when I dug into my strawberry shortcake, there was a pear-shaped diamond!"

One woman I know posted a calendar on the refrigerator door with her deadline for her live-in partner to propose, as if it were a "Things to Do" list. Sometimes men do need a kick in the pants, though. I tried giving my fiancé The Deadline a couple of times. He never really took me seriously, and about a week after I had given him The Deadline I would forget the date. Of course, giving a man The Deadline is never a wise idea. Even after the fiancé proposed, though it really was a surprise, I cried, "You really didn't want to, did you? It's only because I practically forced you to propose to me."

"No. You couldn't have made me propose to you. I couldn't be forced into something as serious as this," he had told me. "I proposed because I wanted to." Which made me happy.

I never really thought about having children until I reached age twenty-seven—in fact, I remember feeling the first twinges when I saw a baby right on my twenty-seventh birthday. They were fleeting twinges, but I felt them. But I never felt the urgency to procreate. I had time, I thought. A lot of time. First I had to rule the world. It's the same thing with marriage. I never dreamed about my wedding day when I was a child—to this day I have never dreamed about it. But when I hit twenty-seven, getting engaged suddenly became an absolute necessity, like potato chips after smoking a joint. It was all I could think about. Why hasn't he proposed? When is he going to propose? What is wrong with me that he hasn't proposed? Is he ever going to propose? All around me, everyone seemed to be getting engaged—women *younger* than me, who had been with their boyfriends for much *less* time than I had been with my guy. When the whole world seems to be getting engaged and you're not, you become paranoid that it's never going to happen for you. Which is why you can't help but come up with The Deadline. And then, once he does propose, you put a spin on the memory.

In the same way, I'm going to need a spin on this pregnancy. Instead of "Well, the fiancé and I got looped at our engagement party. Then, in the throes of passion, I begged him to stay in me, and then the idiot did, and now, in a few short months, we're going to have a baby! Hurray for us!" I'll have to say something like "We talked about it and decided we really wanted to get pregnant. It was the right time. We're so in love. It just seemed the right next step!" But in case no one believes that—because nothing that lovey-dovey has ever come out of my mouth—I'm going to say this was a "love child." It *was* a "love child" in the sense that we were very much in love—drunk with love—when the child was conceived. See? It's easy to put The Spin on things that don't go the way we think they are supposed to. Women are geniuses at The Spin.

FEBRUARY 10

Two weeks ago it seemed everyone I knew was getting married, getting pregnant, or having babies. Now that *I* may be pregnant, all the people I thought were married and having babies have disappeared. Where did they all go? I couldn't possibly have imagined all those people, could I?

Not that any of my worries matter now. I woke up with the most painful cramps I have ever had. My period is for sure coming any second. I took three Advils, as I always do when I get cramps, but the pills are not working like usual. In a matter of days, all this worry will be over and I can get on with my life. I can get my relationship back on track. I can get back to work. I can drink again, without worrying that I am going to give birth to a three-headed circus freak because I indulged in a few glasses of wine and a few cigarettes. Why am I not thrilled then? Why does getting my period depress the hell out of me?

There are definitely right reasons and wrong reasons to have a baby. To buy cute baby clothes and shoes is definitely not a right reason to have a baby. Even I know that. How did people have babies before the Internet, I wonder? I found this list on the Net:

RIGHT REASONS TO HAVE A BABY

1. You and your husband have both chosen to do this.
2. You want to start being a giver and stop being a receiver.
3. You are finished trying to achieve your goals in the outside world.
4. You want the challenge of having a baby.
5. You are looking forward to the process of raising a child.
6. You want to give birth as a personal expression of yourself.

WRONG REASONS TO HAVE A BABY

1. So your friends and relatives will stop pressuring you.
2. Because you have a number of friends who are already mothers.
3. To get time off work.
4. To guarantee there is someone to take care of you when you are older.
5. To be adored by another living being.

I hate these lists. Unprepared people don't do lists. It's like whoever came up with this list has never heard of the "unplanned pregnancy" or "pleasant surprise," which I know for a fact happens all the time. I read somewhere that more than 50 percent of pregnancies in the United States are unplanned. It was a relief, for about ten seconds, to know that I wasn't alone. Who wants to stop being a "receiver" all the time? And last time I checked, I haven't won a Nobel Prize for literature, or even received a raise in a while. So, no, I haven't exactly achieved my goals in the outside world just yet, but who has? I'm not sure I'm up for the challenge of having a baby—but who ever is, except maybe Celine Dion? I'm not even sure how giving birth would be a personal expression of myself. And, please, what human in this world does not want to be adored by another living being, does not want time off work? And doesn't everyone worry about being old alone, living with eighteen pet rabbits as their sole companions? I haven't really thought that my baby might adore me. I'm too busy complaining about how the baby is going to ruin my life while hoping the baby can't hear me. What if the fetus already needs therapy? None of that's to say that I couldn't do it. Just because I'm not looking forward to getting fat and can't imagine yelling at a thirteen-year-old to clean his or her room doesn't mean I'm not going to enjoy parenthood, does it?

FEBRUARY 12

7:55 a.m.
Just got my period. I am sure of it . . .

7:56 a.m.
False alarm.

2:00 p.m.
My period just arrived!

2:01 p.m.
False alarm.

4:34 p.m.
I know my period just came. This time it's really
for real. I can feel wetness Down There.

53

4:35 p.m.
False alarm again.

9:00 p.m.
Great. I got my period and just ruined this pair of
DKNY silk pants. I can feel it. This time it's really,
really for real. I am absolutely positive I just got
my period.

11:00 p.m.
Going to bed. I want to be well rested when I visit
the fiancé this weekend. My period did not come.

10:30 a.m.

On a plane, on my way to visit the fiancé for Valentine's Day. I will not ruin this weekend with talk of pregnancy, missed periods, babies, or anything at all that has to do with us being parents in the very near future and our lives changing forever. In fact, I will not even call him "babe." Maybe my period is just late. Or maybe it's not late. Maybe it's not supposed to come until Monday. I'm still not exactly sure what day my period came last month. I just know the exact day I bought tampons. I still have wicked cramps. My breasts are very tender. I really do feel like my period is going to come any second. I have finished the bottle of Advil.

10:00 p.m.

The fiancé took me out for dinner. It was almost like before the maybe-to-a-good-chance-that-he's-knocked-me-up days. He didn't comment when I ordered chicken fingers. The cramps even went away during dinner, but they returned as soon as we got back to his place.

I love the fiancé's condo. It's a bachelor's kind of place. Although there is no bearskin rug or automatic curtain closers or waterbed, it is definitely more Bachelor Pad than Daddy Pad. There is nothing actually living in this place—no plants, no fish, and, thanks to his once-a-week cleaning lady, no mold. It's all mahogany, burgundy, marble, and hardwood. He has the most comfortable king-size bed I have ever been in, and blackout blinds to ensure the best sleep possible. He has a steam shower with ledges you can sit on and a huge whirlpool bathtub he's never used. There are two ovens in the kitchen, which also have never been used. While my place is un-child-friendly because of all the crap and matches and dirty dishes and ashtrays lying around on my floor, his place is equally un-child-friendly because of all the sharp edges and expensive R-rated material—meaning material not meant for sticky children. There's no way he'd allow a dog on his couch or on his 500-thread-count sheets, let alone a pukey baby. I love his place. Visiting the fiancé is like staying at a hotel, minus the room service. A baby in here would be as out of place as a baby in a strip club.

We do not have sex tonight. I tell him I have cramps, which is entirely true. The fiancé believes me, of course, but I don't think that he really believes my period is ever going to come. I know it is. I can *feel* it.

FEBRUARY 16

On the plane heading back home. The weekend was extremely relaxing. We talked about nothing serious. I'm trying not to think about it, but I can't help it: we did not have sex once this weekend. We barely fooled around. The most sexual we got with one another was when I practically forced him to feel me up.

"Do my breasts feel larger?" I asked him. "I think they feel larger. They're definitely more tender. What do you think?"

"I'm not sure," he said. "Don't they always get this way before you get your period?" he asked, taking his hand off my breast. We had been standing in his walk-in closet. Suddenly we are very comfortable with the word "period." Was he trying to reassure me? Or to reassure himself?

"Yeah, I'm supposed to get it any day now. So that's probably right." That was the closest we came to talking about me being pregnant.

If my period doesn't come by tomorrow morning, I'm going out to buy a home pregnancy test. Then I will know.

FEBRUARY 17

11:00 a.m.

In a plastic bag, inside another plastic bag, which is inside my purse, I have the goods. My period never came.

Purchasing the home pregnancy tests was much as you would expect: a less-than-pleasurable experience. I must remember next time (as if!) not to go shopping for a home pregnancy test dressed in baby blue sweats with my hair in a ponytail.

Though I am twenty-nine, even on a good day—a day when I have tried to look like a mature adult—I still get carded for cigarettes and asked for ID when I go to certain bars or to the liquor store. With my hair in a ponytail and wearing baby-colored clothes, I couldn't help but feel the way I probably looked, standing in front of the home pregnancy tests, to the outside world: like an unwed high school student who did something very stupid.

I did not tell the fiancé what I was doing today. I've decided to tell him only after I know for sure.

I had no idea that home pregnancy tests were such a big business. There are dozens and dozens on the shelves. Who made the decision, I wondered, to place the home pregnancy tests on the same shelf as the condoms? As if I didn't already feel silly enough without a box of condoms mocking me.

"Can I help you?" asked the white-haired pharmacist. I had been standing there, in front of the condom/pregnancy-test shelf, for fifteen minutes. There was one thing I needed this pharmacist to know: I desperately needed him to know that I was engaged and not, as he probably assumed, a careless student who had possibly screwed up her life. I needed this pharmacist to know that there was a man out there who loved me enough to ask me to marry him, so it was okay that I was having sex. How do I flash my ring and make it look like nothing out of the ordinary?

"Did you want to purchase some condoms?" he asked.

"Ah, no." Could this possibly get any worse? It's like I was an actor in a bad after-school special. I tried to be clever. "But that would have been great a couple weeks ago." The pharmacist didn't attempt a smile.

"Are all these home pregnancy tests the same?" I asked him, running my left hand, the one with the engagement ring, along the shelf. "There are just so many brands," I mused, continuing to run my hand along the shelf.

"Yes, they are all the same."

I picked out four and walked to the counter.

"So, is this the one you have decided on?" asked the pharmacist, picking up the box closest to him.

"Oh no. I want all four of them."

"You want them all?"

I wondered if I should crack a joke about buying early Christmas gifts for my friends, but, remembering the reaction to my previous attempt to be clever, I concluded that home pregnancy tests were no joke to a pharmacist.

"Yes, yes, I'm going to buy them all."

"Okay," he said, ringing them up. "That will be $92.14."

There is nothing that makes a woman more bitter than spending money on things she doesn't want to spend money on, like toilet paper and toothpaste. These supplies are necessary, but you'd rather spend the money on something frivolous, like a new belt. But considering I had spent $45 on shampoo just two days earlier, I figured this was not the time to start being cheap.

"Can you double bag that?" I asked. I was afraid that I would run into someone I knew. Of course, most people I know—aside from Lena, an aspiring novelist, who works out of her home, as I do—would be at work. But I had lines prepared just in case. "Oh, yes. One of my good friends thinks she might be pregnant," I would say. "Can you imagine? She's too embarrassed to come in here herself, so I offered to do it for her. I'm going to her place now to drop them off." I didn't run into anyone. There was nothing to do but go home, drink some water, and do the test. I mean, *tests*.

I'm not sure why I'm not racing to do the tests. Possibly because the whole experience of buying the tests was so exhausting. Maybe I don't really want to find out. Is it conceivable that I will be disappointed if I haven't conceived? Maybe I do want to be pregnant. One thing is certain: I will feel like a moron if I'm not pregnant, knowing I went through all this drama for nothing. There is one person I need to tell that I am doing the test. It is only right. I call the fiancé. Okay, I lie. I call Lena, the first person I told about my pregnancy.

"Hey, I got the tests," I say when she picks up. I don't even say hi.

"You did?"

"Yes, they're right here. I got four of them."

"You bought four home pregnancy tests? Why? Are you crazy?"

"Well, in my defense, the editor of *Jane* magazine did seven home pregnancy tests. I remember reading that. I think I was being quite good only buying four. Hey, do you want to stay on the phone with me while I do it?"

"Definitely."

While I have a big problem peeing in front of the fiancé, I do not have a problem peeing in front of my girlfriends. Girls pee in front of each other all the time—not just when we go to the bathroom together in restaurants or bars, but when we're at home. We'll take our cells or our cordless phones to the washroom and continue chatting away. You can't put a good conversation on hold for something as mundane as a pee break.

I take Lena to the washroom with me via my cordless phone, giving her a play-by-play of what I'm doing. "Okay, I'm opening the box. Okay, I'm taking the pee stick out of the box. Okay, I'm ready to pee now. Talk to me about something so I don't scare the pee away."

"Um, um, uh. Did you see the latest issue of *Us Weekly*?" Lena asks. "Kate Hudson looks amazing. She looks so much like her mother, it's crazy."

"Okay, I just peed on it. I hope I did it right. I'm going to flush now and wash my hands. Give me a sec," I tell her, putting the phone down on the side of my bathtub, where I also place the home pregnancy test that I just peed on.

"I'm back."

"How long does it take?" asks Lena.

"I could know within thirty seconds and I'll definitely know by two minutes. That's what it says on the back of the box."

I haven't really read the detailed instruction page inside, opting instead to figure it out myself. I mean, how hard is it to figure out how to pee on a stick?

Before I know it, I'm pacing.

"Do you know," I say to Lena, "that I'm pacing? What's that about?"

"Thirty seconds is definitely up. Go back to your washroom and check!"

"Okay, here I go," I say, taking Lena with me. "OH MY GOD! TWO BLUE LINES! TWO BLUE LINES!"

"OH MY GOD! Wait—what does that mean?"

"I don't know! I don't know! I didn't read the damn instructions!"

"Well, you idiot, read them!"

"Okay, let me look . . . give me a sec . . . Oh. Yup. Two blue lines means . . . I'm pregnant."

"Oh my God. I knew you were."

"What? You didn't believe me when I told you. You said, and I quote, 'You are not pregnant. What are the chances?' I remember you specifically saying, 'You are not pregnant.'"

"I know. I know. But I still knew you were."

61

"You did?"

"Yeah, I just had a feeling."

"You did?" Well, why the fuck didn't she humor me then?

"Well, congratulations."

"Yeah. Thanks, I guess."

"How are you feeling about this all?"

"I think I'm going to be sick."

"Are you going to call the fiancé and tell him right now?"

"Maybe in a bit. I think I'm going to be sick."

"Are you happy, sad, what?"

"I think I'm going to be sick."

"Stop freaking out, Beck. You know, the most surprising people can turn out to be the best mothers."

"You're right. Let's talk later," I say, hanging up.

Wait—the most surprising people can turn out to be the best mothers? What the hell does that mean?

1:00 p.m.

I am not going to call the fiancé at work to tell him the news. First I have to figure out what to say.

1:10 p.m.

Yeah, I really shouldn't call the fiancé at work to tell him. I should wait until he's at home, so as to not disturb him at the office. And definitely until I figure out how to break the news.

1:12 p.m.

Definitely not going to call. Definitely not.

1:15 p.m.

I couldn't help it. I called the fiancé at work to tell him that I did a home pregnancy test and it was positive. Luckily, it went straight to his voice mail. God, apparently, doesn't think I should tell him just yet either. I hung up without leaving a message.

3:00 p.m.

Peed on the second test, waited thirty seconds. It was also positive.

5:30 p.m.

Ditto with the third test. Positive. *Quel surprise!*

8:00 p.m.

The fourth test is positive. I'm starting to believe that I really might be pregnant.

FEBRUARY 18

I've lined up all my positive home pregnancy tests in a row on the bathroom counter. I've memorized the pamphlets, which all pretty much say the same thing: "The test is greater than 99.9 percent accurate. In consumer studies, over 100 participants' results obtained with this test were all correct. In laboratory studies with 298 urine samples, the answers were all correct when compared to tests used in hospital laboratories. You can therefore be confident of getting hospital-quality results at home."

There's no chance that four home pregnancy tests which are 99.9 percent accurate are all wrong, is there?

I call Lena.

"Lena. They're all positive!"

"You did them all?"

"Yes. I stayed in all day yesterday doing home pregnancy tests. They're kind of addictive. I wish I had another one."

"Well, at least you know now for sure, for sure, for sure you're pregnant. Now you have a real reason to freak out and not just a pretend reason, like you usually do."

"Yeah, that's true."

"Hey, you know, you could've done all the tests at the same time. You could have peed on all four sticks in one go."

"Yeah, that's also true. I never thought of that. But isn't it clear? I'm a freaking idiot!"

I call Ronnie too. Does every other woman know what they are supposed to do right after taking a home pregnancy test which turns out to be positive? What are you supposed to do? Ronnie was driving her son to his playgroup or a birthday party or the dentist, *somewhere*. I'm not sure. I really wasn't paying attention.

"I told you. I was right!" I begin.

"Right about what?"

"I'm pregnant. I did four tests and they all came up positive. What do I do now?"

"You did four tests? And they're all positive?"

"Yes! I told you I was pregnant, and remember you didn't believe me? You should really listen to me!"

"I'm sorry, Beck. But I think you also told me you could feel the baby moving inside you three hours after you had sex, which is impossible."

"What do I do now?"

"First, call your doctor. He'll give you a referral to an obstetrician. You have to get one fast. But if you want, you can use mine. He delivered all three of my babies and I love him. I'll call you later to give you his number. And you have to get Materna immediately. And also, you should pick up some pregnancy books. I'll give you a couple of titles that all my pregnant friends swear by. And you have to quit smoking immediately. You're smoking right now! I can hear you inhaling!"

"Ronnie! You're freaking me out. What is Materna?"

"It's a vitamin that has all the vitamins you need in one. It has folic acid in it, which is very important so your baby won't have spina bifida. Go get it right now. If you don't get it by tomorrow, I'm going to drag you to the drugstore and buy it for you."

"Well, can I at least tell the fiancé that I'm pregnant first?"

"You haven't told him yet?"

"Not exactly."

"What do you mean, 'not exactly'? You have to tell him. This is not something you can keep a secret, like the time you returned that bracelet he got you for rent money. He's going to find out."

"I think, in the back of his mind, he already knows."

"You have to get married now too. And learn to cook! And you definitely have to get your driver's license. You can't be a mother without a driver's license."

I love Ronnie, but she made me feel like I have already screwed up this child by not being married, by not having a driver's license, by not knowing what Materna is, by not knowing how to cook. My license was taken away from me after I got three speeding tickets in one week and failed to pay the fine within the six-month period. I obviously was not meant to be a driver. Am I meant to be a mother? Now, along with figuring out how to raise a child and where to get Materna, I also have to get my license back? Why don't I just shoot myself now? I need a drink.

I call Dr. R., who has been my physician for as long as I can remember. I must have called during a slow time because he comes to the phone immediately.

"Hi, Dr. R.," I say. I always get nervous when I

talk to him. I'm not sure why. "I just did a home pregnancy test and it's positive."

Dr. R. tells me I should come to his office for a blood test, which, frankly, is a bit of a pain as his office is quite far from my house.

"Really? Even though I did two home pregnancy tests, which both came up positive?" I don't want to tell him I did four. It now seems a little overboard.

"When was the first day of your last period?" asks Dr. R.

Thank God, I know the answer to this. "January 13th or 14th, around there."

"Well, your period is only a couple of days late then. It could just be your hormones going wonky. You need a blood test. Come in tomorrow morning."

Maybe it really is too soon to tell, 100 percent, if I'm pregnant. Maybe my hormones *are* just wonky. No sense in not having one cigarette. No sense in telling the fiancé until I know not just 99.9 percent, but 100 percent. I'm going to do a blood test tomorrow, and when I get the results back, I'm going to tell the fiancé immediately. That's the plan and I'm sticking to it.

FEBRUARY 19

Of course, plans don't always go according to plan. I told the fiancé that I did a home pregnancy test and was going to my doctor to do a blood test. I couldn't help it.

"I did a home pregnancy test this morning," I lied, calling him, exactly as I said I wouldn't do, at his office. He doesn't need to know that it was done yesterday.

"Let me guess. It was positive, right?" This is why the fiancé gets paid the big bucks. He knows what's going on.

"It was."

I heard him sigh. I don't like it when the fiancé sighs. When he sighs, it usually means he's frustrated or, worse, that I've done something wrong.

"But," I said, hopefully, "I called my doctor and he said that it could be just my hormones going wonky because it's really too soon after I missed my period to know anything for sure. I'm going there tomorrow," I lied again. I was actually heading to see Dr. R. in twenty minutes, but I needed to buy myself some time to think. "Then we'll know for sure."

"How long until you get those results back?"

"He said two days at the most. Don't worry. What are the chances?"

The fiancé responded by sighing.

I have put the four home pregnancy test pee sticks in my desk drawer. I am pretty sure this is completely unsanitary. I don't care. I want to keep them, no matter how gross it is. I'm only going to be pregnant once, after all.

4:00 p.m.

Just picked up my home messages. I actually managed to do a couple of interviews today, and to
write a feature. I feel very accomplished. And at
least readers will know everything about married
women hiding secret credit cards from their husbands. They shouldn't be punished just because
I'm going through all this.

A sexy new intern showed up at the office today.
Word is Sexy Young Intern looks like a twenty-
year-old Sophia Loren, and she's also been put on
the Young Hip beat. *My* beat. Is it possible my boss
is already looking for a flat-stomached, non-
pregnant replacement for me? Oh God, men *love*
Sophia Loren. *Women* love Sophia Loren.

And then . . .

"Hi. It's Dr. R. Your blood work came back. It's
definitely positive. Call me to talk about what you
want to do next."

I listen again. "Hi. It's Dr. R. Your blood work
came back. It's definitely positive. Call me to talk
about what you want to do next." And one more
time. "Hi. It's Dr. R. Your blood work came back.
It's definitely positive. Call me to talk about what
you want to do next." I save the message. It turns
out that I am super fertile and that the fiancé has
supersperm. It turns out that you can get knocked
up after only one time without protection, no
matter how much you had to drink beforehand. It

turns out that no matter how unprepared you are to be pregnant and raise a child, you can still get pregnant. God, I really do not want to get fat. I must remain skinny like Sexy Young Intern. And, yes, that's really on my mind.

11:00 p.m.
"Hi. It's Dr. R. Your blood work came back. It's definitely positive. Call me to talk about what you want to do next." I couldn't help it. I had to hear it just one more time.

It's not that the fiancé and I have never discussed having children. If you're in a relationship and a number of your couple friends start getting pregnant, you're kind of forced to have the discussion. But the fiancé has always said, "Children are for life," and "We have to live together before we have a child," and "I'm not sure why anyone has children." Which is why I don't think the fiancé is going to be thrilled when he finds out he's going to be a father in eight months. While I have always known the fiancé is "father material," he doesn't seem to know it. I don't know much about parenting, but I'm sure raising a child would be much better if the father was into it and not all like, "I'm not sure why anyone has children." Unfortunately, when the fiancé talks about being a parent, he makes it sound like such a downer. I have to admit, I see his point. Whenever I see a mother trying to calm her baby down in a restaurant or trying to shut it up in a grocery store, or especially on an airplane, I'm not sure why people have children either. Once you have a child, it *is* forever.

I have to tell the fiancé. I will, first thing tomorrow.

2:00 a.m.

I can't stop thinking about what has gone into my body over the past few weeks.

THINGS I HAVE DONE THAT COULD ALREADY
HAVE SCREWED UP MY UNBORN CHILD

1. Numerous cosmopolitans on night of conception
2. Entire bottle of Advil since conception
3. Maybe five glasses of wine
4. Twenty-one cups of coffee
5. A few tablespoons of NyQuil
6. A dozen or so chocolate bars
7. A dozen or so spin classes
8. One hair coloring
9. Numerous bad thoughts
10. Nightly hot baths
11. Cigarettes
12. Sushi

THINGS I KNOW I HAVE NOT DONE
THAT COULD HURT MY BABY

1. Heroin
2. Bounced on a trampoline

I told the fiancé. I just came out and said it. "The blood test came back positive."

I told him we couldn't tell anyone just yet because it's very early and we have to figure out what we want to do. I did not tell him that Lena and Ronnie and Dana already knew. I had a solid list of arguments prepared. I was going to say something like "I've really thought about this. I'm not too young to have this child. It's my choice, and if you don't want to participate in the raising of this child, that is your choice and I will be okay with that. I will do it on my own. I will still love you, and I totally understand." Of course, I would totally *not* understand. I'm a little disappointed that I didn't get to use any of my prepared speech. I didn't even get to use my favorite line: "I know this isn't the ideal time. But, really, when would be the ideal time to have a baby?" I don't actually remember what the fiancé said in response to my news. I know there were sighs. I know there were no tears, of sadness or of joy. I've never seen the fiancé cry anyway.

He's decided to come visit me next weekend so we can talk about all this in person. The good news is he didn't demand I get an abortion and he didn't say anything about breaking up with me. Unless, of course, he's going to break up with me in person! Which is, technically, better than ditching me over the phone. After five years in a relationship, a person deserves to be broken up with in person.

The unfortunate thing about knowing you are pregnant almost the second it happens is that you have to keep the secret for so long. It would have been so much better, I think, to not have known for at least a couple of months. I've heard stories of women who didn't realize they were pregnant until they were in their fifth month. I am super jealous of these women, who could go on with their lives—drinking and partying—for more than half their pregnancies without consciously knowing they could be harming their offspring. I want to be one of *those* women. Instead, I worry that maybe something is going to go wrong and I'll miscarry, which is even more depressing than knowing I'm pregnant. Already every time I go to the washroom I can't help but look down to see if there is the slightest trace of blood on the toilet paper, proof that something may be going wrong. Ten percent of women miscarry in their first three months of pregnancy, I learned through my Internet research. I can't think of anything worse than telling everyone I know that I'm pregnant only to miscarry two weeks later. Which is the real reason I told the fiancé we couldn't tell anyone yet. I have already decided to keep this child, God help us all, but I am definitely not going to tell anyone until the three-month mark, which is in about sixty days. I still can't believe that my period isn't

coming. Women's intuition, four home pregnancy tests, and one blood test pretty much convince you that you are indeed pregnant. But for
some reason it still feels as though my period is
about to arrive any second.

I can do it. I can keep a secret for sixty days. I
know I can. Easy. I am also going to quit smoking
now that I know I'm pregnant. Right after this last
goodbye-to-smoking cigarette. Quitting is going
to be super easy now that I know I'm harming
someone else's lungs and not just my own.

FEBRUARY 22

I woke up with a wicked sore throat today. I think I
have a fever. I need antibiotics *right now.* I know I
do. I have always been a bit of a pill popper—not
in a Stepford Wives kind of way, but when I feel
the slightest headache coming on, I will take three
Advils. For years, Advil has been my best friend.
If I was wearing uncomfortable high heels—the
kind of heels that are for standing around in, not
walking around in—I would pop Advil before
heading out for the night. Advil preempts the
pain of wearing standing-only shoes. I would pop
three Advils before getting bikini waxes, for the
same preemptive powers. I have never been a
good sleeper, so I often take sleeping pills—
prescription, over-the-counter, the ones my
friends get from their doctors and share with me,

whatever. I will even take NyQuil, for that woozy high it gives you right before you fall asleep. I live for that dreamlike state. I know I can't take any of that anymore.

I called Ronnie to ask her what I can do about my sore throat. The conversation was short. She was entirely unhelpful.

"Ronnie, I have a sore throat. What can I take?"

"Nothing."

"But, can I at least—"

"No!"

"Can I have some—"

"No!"

"Should I call my doctor?"

"Don't bother."

"Do you really think if I just took one—"

"NO!"

"So you're telling me I can't take anything?"

"NO! I mean, yes. Yes, you can't take anything at all now that you're pregnant."

"Are you sure I can't even—"

"NO!"

And that's pretty much how it went.

How does one get better without taking some sort of medication or popping some sort of pill? That's, like, *unheard* of.

8:00 a.m.

I have never been much good at keeping secrets. My friends will say, "Can you keep a secret?" as they lean in to tell me something juicy. And I will say, "Of course," but really I can't. Few people are really good at keeping secrets. But I'm going to be this time. To keep my mind off this huge secret I am keeping, I am going to the bookstore. Pregnancy reading should keep me busy and my mouth shut. My throat is still sore and I have the sniffles. I think I'm allergic to being pregnant.

Noon

Well, maybe I should at least tell my mother the news. She is my mother, after all. And I feel like I need my mommy right now, as though I fell off my bike and the only one who can make it better is her. I really do want to tell her, but I can't get the thought out of my mind that telling your parents you're pregnant is admitting to them you've had sex, and not very careful sex at that. My parents and I do not have that kind of relationship. We do not talk about sex at the dinner table. I still remember the one sex talk they had with me. I was about sixteen and doing homework when there was a knock at the door. Two minutes before, I had heard the same knock on my older brother's door. They entered my room hand in hand. "We just want you to know there are a lot of bad diseases out there," said my mother, my father nodding silently by her side. I knew immediately this was a talk about condoms. "Um, okay," I responded. "Thanks, I know." I was a couple of years away from having sex anyway. I didn't even have a first boyfriend yet. Then my parents left my room, hand in hand. And that was that. That was the extent of my sex talk. Quick and easy.

I decided to pick up the phone and call my mother anyway. It was time to tell her that her daughter was no longer a virgin.

"Mom," I began. "I have some news. I'm pregnant."

"What? When did you find out?"

"Yesterday. I went to see Dr. R."

"Ahhh. That's so great. Congratulations. I'm so happy for you. Are you getting married now?"

I couldn't deal with the when-are-you-getting-married lecture right now. "I guess we will. Maybe in the summer."

My mother was clearly happy, probably because she could boast to all her friends that she was, finally, going to be a grandmother. For most mothers of adult children, this is a big deal.

"You can't tell anyone yet," I told her. "I'm only like a month pregnant. We have to wait until I'm three months, okay?"

"Okay, you tell me when it's okay."

The strangest thing, though—my father didn't come to the phone, nor did he call me later. Perhaps it's harder for fathers to accept the fact that their daughters have sex than it is for mothers. Who knows.

There is one other relative who will need to know: my ninety-year-old grandfather. No sense in telling him just now. He's a pretty hip and happening man for ninety, but I don't think he'll approve of the whole getting-pregnant-before-marriage thing. I'm going to wait a bit before giving him his first heart attack.

FEBRUARY 24

I think my friend Vivian is pregnant. It takes one pregnant gal to recognize another. Vivian is thirty-five and has been married for about four months to a lovely man named Donald.

Shannon, Heather, Vivian, and I met at a hotel bar for an after-work drink today. I couldn't drink, but I am not going to change my routine just because I'm pregnant. I'm still going to be a hip woman who hangs out at hip hotel bars, bump or no bump. I just won't drink. Except for Perrier.

"What can I get you?" asked the surly waitress. You have to love hotel bars, with the middle-aged waitresses and the free nuts on the table.

"I'll have an orange juice," Vivian said, which I immediately found odd. It was 5:30.

"I'll have a glass of your house red," said Shannon.

"I'll have the same. Red wine," said Heather.

"Um, I think I'll just stick to Perrier," I told the waitress. I glanced at my friends, who, as I suspected, were looking at me in disbelief. "I'm not feeling so well today," I said, defensively. Why am I defending myself? Can't I not drink in front of them? Is that so wrong?

They didn't seem to give Vivian the same look. Maybe they all knew something I didn't.

Shannon and I, who live in the same area, shared a cab ride home, while Vivian and Heather walked to their homes.

"Shannon, is Vivian pregnant?" I asked.

"How did you know? But you can't tell anyone! She's almost at three months, but she's not telling anyone until then." See? I told you none of my friends could keep secrets.

"I just assumed, because she was drinking orange juice at six o'clock in a hotel bar. That's such great news for her."

"Yeah, I'm so happy for them. But you weren't drinking either. What's up with that?"

"Well, it's not because I'm pregnant. It's because I'm not feeling well and need a little break from booze." I could see how the next few weeks were going to be for me—lies, lies, and more lies.

FEBRUARY 27

The fiancé is coming to visit tomorrow. This week, a new fear entered my mind: I started to worry that the fiancé is going to think I tricked him into getting me pregnant. I didn't. I just asked—rather, I begged—and he did. But still, occasionally in the past, my friends and I have joked about gals tricking guys into getting them pregnant. We joke about this in the same way we joke about our Plan B's.

Having a Plan B is just good sense for women. What could be worse than to hit forty with no boyfriend and no sperm at your disposal just as your maternal clock is running out of juice? Having a Plan B ensures that this never happens. Shannon, Heather, Lena, and I spend a lot of time talking about the successful women we know who own their own homes, who have done wonders in their careers, but who have no family. We all agree that there's something very depressing about this. I once left a job because I was working with a number of women ranging in age from thirty-five to fifty, not one of whom was in a serious relationship. Not one of those women had any children. They all worked twelve-hour days, and I used to sometimes wonder, Is this God's way of showing me what the future has in store for me? So I quit.

My Plan B—which it seems is now obsolete—was my high school boyfriend, whom I dated for three years. He would have been a good sperm donor for the same reasons he was a good high school boyfriend: he has green eyes, curly hair, and musical talent. Our child would not only have been incredibly cute, but would have had a singing voice to die for. When I asked him a few years back if he would be willing to be my Plan B, he agreed eagerly. If I reached age thirty-five—my personal scary age—and didn't have a man in my life to be the father of my child, he would have sex with me. But maybe he was just agreeing because he wanted to have sex. He would probably make an awful father. But that's not something I worried about. He was just a Plan B, after all. No woman actually believes she will ever have to resort to *using* her Plan B.

FEBRUARY 28

5:00 p.m.

There are things I know about babies and a lot of things I do not know about babies. I know that I do not like sitting beside babies on airplanes. I know that I do not like sitting near babies in restaurants. I know that I want to yell at people who bring babies into movie theaters. But I do not know how to hold a baby. In fact, I have never held a baby. I do not know how to change a baby or how to feed a baby.

So, while waiting for the fiancé to arrive, I decided to flip through some of the pregnancy books I picked up the other day, so I can at least know something about being pregnant. The books were still in the bag, lying by my front door where I had dropped them. Obviously, I wasn't as curious as I thought I'd be to find out what happens during pregnancy. Which is surprising. The only thing I know less about than babies is pregnancy.

6:00 p.m.

My God! Instead of using cutesy titles for pregnancy books, why don't they just title them *101 Ways You Can Fuck Up Pregnancy*? Or *101 Things That Can Go Horribly Wrong During Pregnancy*? Or *101 Ways to Harm Your Baby*, or *101 Things You Can't, Under Any Circumstances, Do While Pregnant*, or *101 Ways Your Body Will NEVER Be the Same*? Awful, awful, awful things happen to a woman's body when she's pregnant. All the books keep welcoming me to "the mommies' club" and to this "wonderful, joyous" time, demanding that I "enjoy every minute of this miracle." How can any woman possibly enjoy the miracle of pregnancy once she finds out all the ghastly things that are about to happen to her body? As if gaining so much weight wasn't awful enough, I learned about hemorrhoids, uncontrollable gas, and hair that grows on places that hair should *never*, ever grow. I hadn't even known what hemorrhoids were. There are some things that no person should ever have to learn about. Hemorrhoids are definitely one. Flipping through those books was a big mistake for so many reasons.

I bought four books because I had bought four home pregnancy tests and thought I should have at least as many books. The first book I picked up had a catchy title. But before I even made it to the first chapter, I knew it wasn't for me. The author, who already had four children and a husband, dedicated the book to her four kids—whose names all began with the same letter. Still, I began reading. It was a book that came highly recommended by Ronnie, after all. I threw the book down in disgust at page 22 after reading, "Sleeveless and pregnancy don't mix" and "By throwing out all your sleeveless shirts, you will be gaining useful drawer space for your nursing bras and giant underwear." Who is this author, with the four children whose names begin with the same letter, kidding? I have never worn giant underwear. I will never wear giant underwear. I decided to wear only tank tops and thongs for the next eight months. I also decided never to open that book again.

One of the co-authors of the second book I picked up gave birth eighteen years ago, which means I am closer in age to her child than I am to her. When this author was giving birth, I was eleven. This, I thought to myself, will be like taking advice from my mother. I gave it a chance. "The results are back," it begins. "Excitement is growing. So is your list of concerns. Will my age or the baby's father's age have an effect on my pregnancy and on our baby? How about chronic medical problems or family genetic problems?" Jesus. I hadn't even thought about that stuff. The author is right, though. I *do* have growing concerns. But they mainly have to do with whether my child will get my nose and my personality. I can't have that. I want my baby to be smart and laid-back, like its father. But I do not want my child to get his hairy back. The child can have my skin and my hair. The child can have his eyes, but not his eyesight. I put the book down.

The third book I flipped through is filled with questions from concerned pregnant women. "I became pregnant again just ten weeks after I delivered my first child. What effect will this have on my health and on the baby I'm now carrying?" And "I'm pregnant for the sixth time. Does this pose any additional risk for my baby or for me?" None of these women ask the questions that haunt me, like "How long before my pants don't fit?" and "How long after I give birth will it take for my pants to fit again?" and "Exactly how fat will I get?" and "Is it wrong to ask the father of my child 1,735 times a day if I'm fat?"

The fourth book I perused is a little too scientific for me. I did learn, though, that the most common concern brought to doctors by pregnant women is alcohol and if the few glasses of wine enjoyed before finding out they were pregnant could have harmed the baby. I learned that after the first month, the baby in my stomach is a tiny tadpole-like embryo, smaller than a grain of rice. Though far from looking human, the tadpole already has a head with a mouth opening, a primitive heart that has begun to pump, and a rudimentary brain, and arm and leg buds will appear soon. There was something about the word "bud" that kind of made me sick. I mean, it's just so freaky weird.

I put the book down and instead decided to watch television to kill time before the fiancé arrives. I wonder if I can go through my entire pregnancy without ever finding out what exactly the placenta is. Or, for that matter, where the uterus is. I think it's entirely possible. I am never studying another pregnancy book again until I absolutely have no choice. It will be just like high school. When I start having contractions, I'll cram.

MARCH 2

6:15 p.m.

The fiancé just left. The fiancé has not reacted to this pregnancy with glee, excitement, or anger, but I expected as much. The fiancé's favorite word to describe pretty much anything and everything is "fine." He could have just eaten the best dinner of his life, prepared by the most talented chef in the world, but ask my fiancé how dinner was and he'll answer, "Fine." His stock could go up $10 in one day, but ask him how this makes him feel and he'll answer, "Fine." He could go on the most exotic, relaxing vacation of his life, but ask him how his week went and he'll answer, "It was fine." So, I suppose, if you were to ask him how he's feeling about impending fatherhood, he'd most likely answer, "Fine." It's not exactly how most women would hope the father of their child would react to such big news. But "Fine" is better than "Fuck. That sucks!" "Fine" is fine by me.

We actually had a pretty relaxing weekend, all things considered. This morning, over eggs Benedict for me and a cheese omelette for him, was really the first time we discussed the pregnancy in great detail. Well, not *great* detail. But some detail. We're moving in the right direction. The fiancé has decided that we, in his words, "have to get our shit together." I agree. We do have to get our shit together. We have about seven months to get off our asses and get our shit together. There is nothing like a deadline to force people to get moving. We have decided that I should probably have the baby in his city. My job allows me to work pretty much anywhere as long as there's an outlet to plug in my computer. It's much easier for me to take a laptop in the overhead baggage compartment than it is for him to pack up his law office. We have also decided, however, that I will keep my apartment so that I can come back whenever I want. After all, my life, my friends, and my family are here.

"We have to get our shit together," he said.

"Yes, let's do that," I agreed. "Let's get our shit together."

"I've already talked to a real estate agent who will let me know about good houses that are coming onto the market." Apparently, getting our shit together for him means house hunting. "And we definitely need a nanny," he continued.

"Definitely."

"And we'll get a night nurse too, for the first couple of months."

"And she can teach me how to take care of a baby, because I certainly don't know a thing about babies."

"I'm quite aware of that. You're a child."

Right. We know.

"Do we really need a house so fast? I mean, don't you think that's too much of a change, too fast? What's wrong with your condo?" I asked him.

"Beck, babies are loud. They cry. And we've never really lived together before. We don't want to be on top of each other. You're going to want your space. And I'm going to want mine."

"But babies are, like, this small," I said, holding out my hands inches apart. "And babies, for the first little while, don't really do anything. They just kind of lie there and sleep, don't they? We have time to buy a house. Do you even have money for a house? I think I have $600 in my bank account."

"Don't worry about it," he said. "Where do you want the nanny and night nurse to sleep? My place is too small for all of us. We definitely need something bigger."

"What about your spare room? We'll just move the desk and computer and the couch into a corner.

Families of four have been known to share apartments smaller than your condo."

"Do you really want to hear the kid screaming all night in the next room? No, we have to get our shit together, and we definitely have to get a bigger place."

"We can put the kid in the crib out in the hallway," I suggested.

"Great. You want to put our child out in the hallway. That's nice."

"I was kidding!"

"Beck, this is not like planning our engagement party. You cannot get bored of being pregnant or get bored of being a mother. This is for the rest of our lives."

God, what does he take me for?

"I know that," I responded. "I am not going to get bored. I promise."

The fiancé is going to send me a plane ticket so I can visit him in a couple of weeks. We might even go look at houses. God, a new house? Living with the fiancé? A baby? All at the same time? It's like . . . it's like I'm a grown-up now. Could there be anything more depressing?

The good news is we had sex! The best part about being pregnant is that you can do it without protection. What's the worst that can happen? You're already pregnant. The first post-getting-knocked-up sex was very sweet. It was actually a little odd—we barely seemed to touch.

"You know," I told the fiancé, "you can still do it on top of me."

"I can? I don't want to hurt anything."

I knew he cared. We agree that sex without a condom feels so much better. Not that I'm suggesting it or anything—look where it got us! It did, however, remind me of a joke I once heard. A man and his pregnant wife had regular sex all throughout her pregnancy. When their son was born, the father held him in his arms for the first time. The baby looked up at his new father and, without warning, punched him. "See?" said the baby to his father. "Now you know what it feels like to be bonked in the face."

MARCH 3

It's strange, but I really don't feel pregnant. The queasiness I experienced the first week after conception and the queasiness I felt after doing the four home pregnancy tests seem to have disappeared. Now I feel nothing. I certainly don't feel like there are arm, leg, and teeth buds growing inside of me. Shouldn't I be feeling something?

MARCH 4

Still don't feel anything different. None of my editors at work seem to have noticed that there is anything different about me. One of them even complimented me on my story about the search for the perfect invisible deodorant. And, yes, it was an investigative piece. You try to find an invisible deodorant that is actually *invisible*. It's impossible.

I have to work harder than ever now that I've seen Sexy Young Intern's byline in the paper several times. She is not going to get my job. It's never going to happen. Even if I have to bring my laptop into the delivery room and continue working all the way through labor.

MARCH 5

Maybe I'm not pregnant. I really do not feel pregnant.

MARCH 6

9:30 a.m.

I just sent my boss an e-mail that began with "I hate my job" and ended with "I think I'm going to quit." Something snapped when I saw there were a couple of editing mistakes inserted into my copy in this morning's paper. I realized that I really hate my job and never want to go back to work again. I'm actually grateful to be pregnant—now I will have something to do when I'm unemployed.

Quitting will be the best decision I have made in a long time. Not like they need me anyway now that they have Sexy Young Intern, who probably has a stomach you could bounce a quarter off of.

9:37 a.m.

Shit! Okay, I love my job. I really, really do. I don't want to quit! What came over me? I must just be grumpy. I send my boss a suck-up, make-up e-mail: "I'm sorry I sent that earlier e-mail. Please ignore it. I'm not feeling great and haven't been sleeping too well. I really do love my job!"

I haven't told my boss that I am pregnant. I don't want the good assignments to be taken away from me and given to Sexy Young Intern. Occasionally work will send me to Los Angeles and New York to cover film junkets, and I get to interview stars. No, this pregnancy is not going to change anything. Not until I get to interview Johnny Depp. Crap. I might have to tell the boss now, though. Is it better to have him know I'm pregnant so I can get away with my bad behavior than to let him believe I'm losing my mind?

6:00 p.m.

Had to leave my spin class midway through. Something about the smell of sweat in the room was making me sick to my stomach. That's never happened before. Plus I was exhausted. I couldn't pedal for another second. That's never happened before either.

8:00 p.m.

"Hello?"

"Beck, what are you doing? You sound wiped out." It's Lena.

"I don't know what I'm doing. What time is it?"

"It's eight o'clock! Were you sleeping?"

"Yeah. I just passed out in front of the television. I don't know what's wrong with me."

"I do."

"What?"

"Um, you're pregnant!"

Oh. My. God. She's right! The nasty e-mail to my boss? The smell of sweat making me want to puke? The fact that I fell asleep at seven o'clock? The symptoms are here. The symptoms are here! Hallelujah, the symptoms are here! I'm not just going crazy!

MARCH 10

Oh God, are the symptoms ever here. Fuck the symptoms. I was nauseous the entire weekend. I barely got out of bed at all. I do not know how I'm going to work today. How can I get out of writing about the new Avon anti-cellulite cream that's all the rage? I don't want to let my readers down. But all I really want to do is to sleep and to be near a toilet. Fuck cellulite.

More than half of all pregnant women experience morning sickness. And morning sickness happens not only in the morning, but all day and all night long. My friend Vivian, who has now come out of the maternity-clothes closet, calls it "mourning sickness," as in mourning the death of her fabulous life. I've figured out that the only way to not feel nauseous is to stuff my face with food. I am now an unattractive pregnant woman whom you cannot force out of bed, but who will occasionally crawl to the kitchen to stuff cookies into her mouth. I am *not* fabulous. But how can I waste away hours of sleeping when I know these are the last few months of my freedom?

I have decided that, instead of books about pregnancy, *Us Weekly* will tell me all I need to know. I can't get enough of *Us Weekly*, with its stories about "Celebrities and Their Kids." It takes me a minute to remember the names of Ronnie's kids, but quiz me on the names of Madonna's kids (Rocco and Lourdes), Calista Flockhart's adopted son (Liam), Angelina Jolie's adopted son (Maddox), or Sarah Jessica Parker's son (James), and I know them all. Maybe I'll also name my child Maddox. It's a good name. Of course, I know someone whose dog is named Maddox. Can I do that to a child?

MARCH 11

The fiancé and I have been having long phone conversations about what kind of parents we want to be. These conversations usually begin with him saying something like "I don't want this baby to change our lives," and me saying, "Don't worry. This will not change our lives." The problem is that most everybody we know who is married and have kids (meaning most of his friends) have all changed. They no longer go out, and if they do, they have to be back early for the babysitter. They seem to talk only about their kids. It's all kind of depressing. We will never become *one of those couples.* We will never become them.

MARCH 21

Lying about being pregnant is more exhausting than actually being pregnant. For what seems like an eternity now, I've been lying. I actually feel like I'm going to explode if I don't tell people soon.

I went out with the girls tonight—Heather, Lena, and Shannon. Like always, we met at a bar. It's what we do. We then headed to a gallery belonging to a friend of Lena's, where there was a show opening. I had slept for most of the day and could have easily stayed in bed all night. But I am adamant that this pregnancy will not change my life, so I forced myself to shower and get dressed. Just the thought of blow-drying my hair almost made me fall asleep standing up.

I knew I was in trouble when we arrived at the bar and grabbed a table for four. I think it was Shannon who threw out the suggestion that we should all just share a bottle of wine. Of course, everyone but me nodded enthusiastically. I spent most of the night running to the washroom, pouring glasses of wine down the sink so Heather and Shannon wouldn't figure out that I wasn't drinking. But every time I sat back down at the table, another glass of wine would be waiting for me. When the bill came, just before we headed to the gallery opening, I chipped in my $80, thinking, I didn't even drink a sip. This pregnancy is costing me a fortune.

Last week, I met a colleague for a drink. Like I said, it's what we do. The problem when you meet friends for "drinks" in a bar is that you are expected to drink. I am starting to think that most of my friendships are based on alcohol. I wonder why we never seem to go to the movies. I purposely arrived ten minutes early when meeting this colleague. A flat-stomached waitress (all women to me are either flat-stomached or not now) came over to where I was sitting. This is how the conversation went:

Her: "Can I get you something to drink?"

Me: "I'm meeting a friend here in a few minutes. But, listen, I'm going to order vodka cranberry when she gets here, but only give me cranberry soda, okay?"

Her: "So you want a vodka cranberry?"

Me: "No, I'm going to order vodka cranberry, but—whatever you do—only serve me cranberry soda."

Her: "I don't understand." (Duh!)

Me: "I'm pregnant, so I cannot drink. But I don't want my friend to find out that I'm pregnant. That's why I'll be ordering vodka cranberry but I only want you to serve me cranberry soda. Get it?"

Her: "Got it."

This is what I'm forced to do now: lie and deceive. It's taking everything out of me. Really, it is.

I cannot even tell you how many times I've used the "I'm on antibiotics" line, or "I can't drink, I have to get up for a very important business meeting early tomorrow," or "I can't drink, I'm still hungover." I've used those excuses so many times in the past few weeks, I'm even boring myself.

1:00 a.m.

I have to get up and pee. I am so tired. I wonder if I can hold it in. No, definitely can't do that. My bladder feels like it's about to explode.

1:45 a.m.
Pee again. What the hell?

3:00 a.m.
Pee. Again.

4:30 a.m.

Pee again. I am going to kill myself if I don't get
any sleep. I don't want to be pregnant anymore. I
never want to pee again. I am never drinking anything again.

MARCH 25

6:00 a.m.

I have never been so hungry in my entire life. I
need food. I hate being pregnant. There must be
women out there who also hate being pregnant.
Where are these women? How come they aren't
speaking up? Or do you forget the bad stuff—the
nausea, the peeing ninety-six times a day, the ten-
hour naps—once the baby is born? It's kind of like
mothers who say their babies sleep the whole night
through. Not every baby can possibly sleep the
whole night through, which means there are a hell
of a lot of mothers out there who are liars.

I'm not lying. I hate being pregnant. I cannot
function like this. I bet Sexy Young Intern is
sleeping like a log. Bitch. I bet the fiancé is also
sleeping like a log. Asshole.

11:00 a.m.

When is this going to end? I can't do anything. I
sleep all day. I have to go pee all night. I'm too
exhausted to pick up a hair dryer, let alone go to
the gym. I'm starting to forget things, too. I think

that's what people mean by Baby Brain. Two days in a row, I've been in the shower and put conditioner in my hair. But, for some reason, I forgot step 1: putting shampoo in my hair. Eating makes me nauseous, but not eating makes me more nauseous. If anyone gives me a strange look, or what I perceive to be a strange look, I burst into tears. But what gets me really bitter is the fact that the fiancé has to go through none of this. I am not going to be able to last the day, let alone the next seven months. Why oh why did I ever ask him to . . . in me?

I am convinced I have already gained fifteen pounds. Ronald McDonald and his Big Macs and super-sized fries are the only things that make me happy. I'm like a freaking kid. I've done the research on weight gain. It's one of the first things I looked up. The average woman usually gains three to four pounds in total during the first trimester and about a pound a week during the second trimester, for a total of twelve to fourteen pounds. During the seventh and eighth months, she'll still gain about one pound per week, but in the ninth month, she'll only gain a pound or two—or even none—for a total of eight to ten pounds during the third trimester. Clearly, I need a calculator. But I think that works out to be somewhere between twenty-five and thirty pounds. I know I have already gained that much. Suddenly I have no willpower when it comes to carbohydrates.

I got mad at Dana yesterday when she called to tell me she feels terrible because she's been to the gym only four times this past week.

"Don't even talk to me about it. I haven't been forever. I miss the gym. I miss my old life." I had, of course, told Dana I was pregnant. Once you share a worry of pregnancy, you have to follow through.

I have no discipline. If I am what I eat, then I'm half McChicken and half Big Mac. I've had three Big Macs in the past week. It's not me who wants McDonald's—it's the baby. You know you're eating far too often at McDonald's when the employees give you a nod of recognition when you are in line. It's happened. Twice. Even though this thing is growing in me, sometimes I wonder if it's indeed my child. This baby wants only white bread and cheese and french fries. Why is the baby doing this to me?

I wonder if Reese Witherspoon ate Big Macs? I wonder if Elizabeth Hurley couldn't stand the smell of salad, let alone eat it? How can I be healthy if everything that is nutritious makes me want to heave?

Thank God the fiancé is coming to visit this weekend. He will not allow me to eat McDonald's.

I'm not sure how he's getting on with "getting his shit together." I have started to get mine together, though. I have paid off my American Express card. I have bought the best hair straightener on the market. It's more important than ever, I figure, that my hair looks good for the fiancé as my ass gets bigger and wider. At least one part of my body should look halfway decent. I made a manicure and pedicure appointment. I made a dentist appointment. Getting my shit together and being responsible is really very tiring. It's enough to make me want to put down this Big Mac and take a nap. No, I'll finish the Big Mac first and *then* take a nap.

MARCH 29

I think this pregnancy thing might actually be sinking in for the fiancé. While we were in a taxi today, he even asked me how I was feeling. Actually, what he said was "Are you going to puke? Because tell me if you are, and I'll tell the driver to pull over." I knew he cared.

But he did get frustrated with me earlier in the day. I had simply asked one tiny little question.

"Does my ass look fatter?"

"No, it's the same as always."

"Take a really good look."

"It's fine." Fine? Fine? How can my ass look just *fine*?

"How about my thighs? I think my pants are a bit tighter around my legs. Do I have fat thighs now?"

"NO!"

"How about my face? Does my face look fatter?"

"Beck, really. Enough already. Your face is not fatter."

"Okay. I'm going to leave you alone." Thirty seconds later I couldn't help myself, though.

"One more question," I said to him.

"What?"

"Are you absolutely, positively sure I'm not fatter anywhere?"

"Yes, I am absolutely, positively sure you are not any fatter anywhere."

"Okay, I promise to leave you alone now."

Of course, I couldn't. I still wasn't sure he was telling the truth.

"One more thing."

"What?!"

"Do you promise to love me forever and ever even when I do get fatter?"

"I promise to love you forever and ever if you just shut the hell up already."

Fine then. You just had to say so. Dealing with me now is nothing. Just wait until I'm in my seventh month.

I also feel like I have to explain myself to the fiancé. We haven't had sex and he's been here two nights. Maybe that's why he hasn't been a willing participant in any of my fat conversations. I can pretty much guarantee we will not be doing it tonight, either, and he leaves tomorrow morning. Because we don't live together, we should technically be having a heck of a lot of sex when we are together, but I am simply not up for it. My "mourning" sickness seems to come on strongest at night.

Not that he wants to have sex with me, either—I haven't been the nicest or easiest person to be around this weekend. I keep making him fetch things for me. How often is too often to use the "I'm pregnant!" line on the father of your child? "Can you get me an orange? I'm dying for an orange. But I feel too sick to get out of bed to get it myself. Please?" And because he is a good, kind man, and because I am pregnant, he will. "Can you peel it for me too? It just tastes better when you peel it for me. And I'm pregnant," I'll whine. I wonder, however, when he'll catch on that mostly I'm just lazy.

So I felt I needed to say something before he goes back home and finally realizes that his secretary is actually pretty hot. "I'm really sorry I don't feel like having sex," I said to the fiancé. "I'm just feeling so tired and bloated and yucky. Don't hate me. Please don't hate me."

"I would never hate you. It's okay. I understand that you are not feeling well."

I'm too tired even to attempt to give him a blow job. If I were a really nice fiancée, I'd at least do that.

I had hoped to save the next little piece of information I threw out to him, but I felt so guilty about not being very affectionate with him all weekend and about his leaving tomorrow that I decided not to wait.

"You know, in the fourth and fifth month of pregnancy, I'm going to be all over you. I'm supposed to get really, really horny then. I'll make it up to you tenfold in a couple of months."

I think he said something like "I can't wait." I'm not sure, though. I had already started to fall asleep.

APRIL 1

I am fat already. I'm convinced the fiancé is going to start having an affair with his secretary. I know it. I just know it. I'm going to be stuck at home, big, fat, and ugly, in a city where I have no friends, and he's going to be getting it on with his blond bombshell of a secretary on the desk at his office. Okay, I don't know for sure that his secretary is blond or a bombshell, or if his desk is even big enough to have sex on. But she probably is sexy.

I had to check. He's back at work now, so I called him at his office.

"Hey, is your secretary blond?"

"Beck, is that you?"

"Yes. Is your secretary blond?"

"What are you talking about?"

"Listen, just answer the question. Is. Your. Secretary. Blond?"

"No, my secretary is not blond."

Oh.

"Well, is she sexy?" It was very important. Yet, somewhere in the back of my mind, I thought,

This really isn't me asking. This is Pregnant Me asking. This is a whole other me. A new me he will just have to learn to love.

"You have nothing to worry about. You're way better looking."

"So you're not going to have an affair with her or anything, right?"

"God. Where do you come up with these things?"

"I don't know. I just do. Do you hate me now?"

"No, I don't hate you. But I have to get back to work. Is that okay?"

"I knew it. You hate me."

In less than two weeks, I can tell people. Hurray! It's probably the pressure of keeping this secret that's turning me into a wacko.

APRIL 4

Again, eleven o'clock on a Thursday night and, professing a headache, I've left Heather, Lena, and Shannon at the bar. When you're the only one not drinking among a group of friends who are, it's not nearly as much fun. Cranberry and soda, or orange juice and soda, or Perrier with lime just doesn't have the same effect as, let's say, a mojito.

Because Lena is the only one who knows about my "condition," she has been helping me out when we go out with Shannon and Heather.

"I'm going to pour my wine into your glass

when you're empty, okay?" I whispered into her ear when Heather and Shannon weren't watching. This was our backup plan. The original plan—for Lena to order for us, out of earshot of anyone else—had failed miserably. Lena ordered a cranberry soda for me, but the bartender handed the happy-colored drink over in a glass as big as the glasses they serve fountain Coke in at Pizza Hut. Apparently when you order Pregnancy Punch in a bar, they serve it in the biggest mother of a glass possible.

"Beck," said Shannon, taking in the colossal cup, "I think the bartender screwed up your order. That is definitely *not* cranberry vodka." When it comes to ordering alcohol, my friends are geniuses.

"I think you're right. Idiot bartender. I think I'll go back up and order a glass of wine. They can't screw that up."

Which is when the backup plan came into effect. It also went disastrously wrong, because Lena, who gets drunk on half a glass of wine, was now drinking both my wine and hers. When Lena started showing off her ability to do backflips in the bar, I knew it would be best for everyone if I just left.

APRIL 5

Noon

"Oh God, I have The Fear," said Lena when she called. She didn't even say hello. "We can't, under any circumstances, do that anymore. I cannot be a trough for your wine. I think I was doing backflips last night. Was I? Was I?"

"Yes, yes, you were. But don't worry. You were pretty good. I had no idea you were that flexible. It's amazing you're still single."

"It *is* amazing I'm still single. But, seriously, I don't want to wake up hungover ever again. I can't do it. I'm going to turn into an alcoholic and end up in rehab. You're just going to have to think of another way to hide that you're not drinking."

"Fine. I will. I think people are on to me anyway." Like most women around age thirty, my friends, like me, have become increasingly suspicious of anyone we know who has recently jumped on the sobriety bandwagon.

"Shannon and Heather asked me point-blank the other night if I was pregnant," I said.

"They did? What did you say?"

"What could I say? I kind of just laughed and said no."

"When are you going to start telling people?"

"Really soon. In just over a week. If I can last."

"If you can last? What about me? I'm a drunk now because you got knocked up!"

It's all about Lena, after all. Not about poor, pregnant, unwed, not-allowed-to-drink, I-don't-know-how-I'm-going-to-get-through-this me.

4:00 p.m.

My breasts are giving me away.

"Did you get a boob job?" asked Helena, my aesthetician, today, when I went in for an underarm wax. "Your breasts are massive!"

"Do I look like the type of woman who would get a boob job?" I responded. "Make that, do I look like the type of woman who could afford a boob job?" I said as I handed her a fistful of quarters for a tip.

In the end, I had to tell Helena the truth. You can't hide anything from your aesthetician. It's like an unwritten rule or something. After all, the woman who gets closest to your private parts is one of the closest women in your life. Not telling the truth to your aesthetician would be like lying to your priest.

"Wow. They are really, really, really big," she said.

"Okay, enough! Leave me and my melons alone. Stop staring! You're making me feel uncomfortable."

The truth is, I can't stop staring at my breasts either. They are fantastic. The one downside is that there are two types of men in this world: Breast Men and Ass Men. The fiancé is an Ass Man. He doesn't appreciate big boobs. So, for the first time in my life, I have big breasts and no one in my life to appreciate them. Except Helena, which doesn't really count. Still, I love my new breasts. They are fabulous. I want to keep them forever and ever. Maybe I should start saving for a boob job.

Suddenly everything has to do with babies. All around me is talk of babies, babies, babies. Is this a new development? Or is it like when you cut your hair to have bangs and you start noticing every other woman out there with bangs?

I was at a house party last night when my good friend Marci, who is a producer on the six o'clock news for one of the main networks, pulled me aside. I consider her my "smart friend," meaning I never willingly get into discussions about politics or fuel emissions with her. But I was more than happy to be dragged away from everyone else I knew. Maybe I'm being paranoid, but I am convinced that all my friends are now paying way too much attention to what I'm drinking—or, rather, not drinking. I was holding a glass of untouched red wine. Just a few more days, I thought to myself. Just hold off a few more days.

"Come with me to get my coat," Marci said to me.

"Wait, are you leaving already?" I asked. I had just arrived.

"Just come with me."

We headed upstairs to the main bedroom, where people had piled their coats on the bed.

"I just needed to tell someone," she said, "that I am s-o-o relieved."

"About what? What's going on?"

"I just got my period."

"Okay, so?"

"Well, remember that guy I went to visit in L.A. a couple months ago?"

Of course, I remembered. Marci had met a guy at a party who was living in L.A. He had invited her down to visit him for a weekend. She had been super excited. But after having an incredible first night with him—meaning they had great sex—he broke it to her that he was interested in someone else. We had long conversations following that weekend, about how a man can sleep with you while being interested in someone else, how men generally have a talent for breaking up with you at the most inappropriate and impolite times. It was almost as bad as being ditched on Valentine's Day or your birthday.

"Well, we weren't so careful. And my period was almost a month late! I just got it here, tonight."

I wasn't sure how to respond. I was relieved because she was relieved. But at the same time, she seemed kind of down.

"Would it have been the end of the world if you had found out you were pregnant?" I asked her.

"Well, that's the thing. I was thinking about it, of course, because I was so late. If I had been pregnant, I probably would have had the baby. I think I could have done it on my own."

At this point I knew I had to fess up about what was going on in my life.

"I have to tell you something, Marci. I'm pregnant."

"You are?"

"Yes, but please don't tell anyone just yet. I'm planning to next week."

"I won't. I promise! This is so exciting," she screeched, giving me a bear hug. Marci is a good friend.

"Are you both just thrilled?"

"Well, it was a bit of a shock, but, yes, we're very happy," I said, saying what you're supposed to say.

"Well, Beck. To tell you the truth, I kind of knew something was up."

"You did? Why? Because I wasn't drinking?"

"No, but the other night when I saw you at Triumph, you were wearing this low-cut shirt and your breasts looked massive. I thought that either you were pregnant or you were PMSing really badly."

I might be able to hide that I'm knocked up, but hiding my knockers is a whole other story. It felt good telling Marci, especially since now I know that even "smart" friends have accidents.

APRIL 7

Before I share my pregnancy with the world—a.k.a. my media friends and my bosses—there was one person I needed to tell first, my Zaida. I got into an argument with my mother over who should tell my ninety-year-old grandfather about the condition I'm now in—meaning the pregnant-without-a-husband condition.

"You tell him," I told my mom.

"No, you tell him. Why should I tell him?" she asked.

"Because he's your father!" I argued.

"But it's *your* baby!" she argued back.

I could see her point. I mean, I am going to be a *mother*. At some point, hopefully sooner rather than later, I am going to have to grow up and do things I don't want to do, like yell at my teenager for stealing the car. But just as I can't see myself doing that, I can't see myself making my grand-father faint either.

"I'm going to call him right now and get it over with," I told my mother.

"You're brave," she said before hanging up.

I knew I definitely had to put a spin on it, for his sake. But I don't think "Hey, Zaida. I'm doing what Elizabeth Hurley, and Rachel on *Friends,* and Miranda on *Sex and the City,* and Madonna, and Julianne Moore, and Goldie Hawn all did—I'm going to have a baby before getting married! Everyone is doing it this way now. Even Colin Farrell has done it this way!" would work.

So instead I called and told him that I had news and that he had better sit down.

"Are you sitting down?" I yelled into the phone. He is ninety, after all.

"No," he said.

"Will you sit down?" I yelled again.

"No."

You can't force a ninety-year-old to do any-thing he doesn't want to do.

"Okay, then. Well, guess what?" I shouted, trying to sound excited. "You're going to be a great-grandfather! Isn't that incredible? You're going to be a great-grandfather," I repeated. I figured that would give him some bragging rights.

"Why? Who's pregnant?" he asked. Maybe I should have been more specific.

"Me! I'm pregnant!"

"Well, how do you like that? Congratulations are in order, I guess. This is happy news, right?"

"Yes, Zaida. It is happy news."

"So are you going to quit work now?" he asked.

"Ah, no, Zaida. Women still work nowadays when they're pregnant, you know."

"So are you getting married now?"

Argh!

Ronnie, my parents, and now my grandfather are all over me to get married. Listening to them tell me to get married just makes me want to go on a long beach vacation. The other day Ronnie insisted again I should be married before giving birth.

"You should get married before you have a baby," she began. "Studies have been done."

"Oh yeah? What studies?"

"Studies showing that children feel more secure when their parents are married. Kids ask questions, you know. One day, your child is going to ask why you and Daddy aren't married or weren't married when she was born."

"Ronnie!" I said in disbelief. When did she turn so, well, *conservative* on me? Is this what having three kids and a husband does to a woman?

"My mother is a teacher. In her class this year there are three students with lesbian mothers! Do you really think it's that important that the fiancé and I don't have a piece of paper saying we're married?"

"Yes."

"Fine. I promise to get married by the time the kid speaks. Wait . . . when do kids start speaking?"

The cold hard truth is that I don't want to get married fat. Now get off my still-bony back.

APRIL 8

Supposedly, or so I've heard, during pregnancy your hair is supposed to get thicker and shinier. I'm still waiting for this to happen. I'm still waiting for my Pantene Pro-V Brooke Shields hair. Supposedly, Sexy Young Intern has great hair. And she's not even pregnant!

APRIL 9

Still waiting . . .

APRIL 10

Still waiting. In fact, I think my hair looks worse than ever, and I suddenly have three pimples. What's the point of being pregnant if your hair looks like crap and you get acne as if you were thirteen again?

APRIL 15

It's time to tell my boss I'm pregnant while assuring him that Sexy Young Intern will not be needed to take over my job. Just because I'm pregnant doesn't mean I'm not cool and hip. I know I'm not the first woman to ever get pregnant, but it feels like I am. Why? Because it's *me* who is pregnant. That's why. But first, I get to tell my friends, which I am looking way more forward to anyway.

APRIL 16

I told Heather, and it was fantastic! There's nothing like flooring your oh-so-cool friends into silence. She was shocked but seemed happy for me. Did I even detect a slight hint of jealousy? There's nothing like having your oh-so-cool friends slightly jealous of you. It doesn't happen very often, so you have to enjoy it when it does.

"Okay, we have to go out and celebrate. Tonight. I don't care what you say," she told me, surprising me with her kindness.

Which is how I ended up telling two perfect strangers and Heather's boyfriend, Charlie, before telling my bosses and most of my friends.

We met Charlie and two of his friends at a restaurant for dinner. I had made Heather "promise" me she wouldn't tell a soul until I had told a few more people myself.

"Have a drink," Charlie and the two other guys, Jim and Seth, kept demanding over dinner. Seth, I noticed, was very cute. Maybe it was just my hormones?

Finally, after the third offer—with much joy because I no longer had to keep the secret—I practically yelled out, "I'm pregnant!"

I pretty much stunned the table into silence. But I got a free dinner out of it because, as they professed, I was now "eating for two." They all kept asking me questions, too, like "How are you feeling?" and "When did it happen?" and "Do you have any cravings yet?" I felt like I was a $1,000 centerpiece at Liza Minnelli's wedding.

Seth, whom I had just met, insisted that they all walk me home after dinner. "You can't walk home alone. You're pregnant." Though I think he really just felt kind of badly for me once he found out that the fiancé was living in a different city. It's okay—I'll take pity. Having people walk you home is better than walking home by yourself.

I tried not to let it bother me that after they all walked me home they were going out to a new club and didn't really invite me. It was like a reverse hostage-taking. I was like, "Please take me!" and they wouldn't. Whatever. I'm pregnant and they're not. What's one night of having friends ditch you?

APRIL 17

The weirdest thing happened. I just received an e-mail from Seth, asking me to go to a movie with him this weekend. I know a flirty e-mail when I receive one. He was flirting. I know it. The strangeness of receiving this e-mail from a cute, single, *employed* male was almost enough to make me forget that I am an unwed, pregnant woman with a fiancé who lives in a different city, a city that I will have to move to even though I have no friends there and it will probably ruin my career and my relationship because the fiancé and I don't even know if we can live under the same roof without killing each other. Almost, but not quite. I had to call Heather to tell her.

"Why do you think he sent me an e-mail asking me to a movie? Don't you think that's a little strange?" I asked her. "I think the guy might actually have a crush on me."

"God, don't even worry about it," said Heather. "Now that you're pregnant, all bets are off. No guy is going to be attracted to you now. No way."

Heather can be malicious sometimes, without thinking about it. Is she trying to tell me, without actually saying it, that her life is more fun because she is *not* pregnant?

But maybe, just maybe, she has a point. There's no way an attractive, single, thirty-three-year-old, *employed* man would ever be attracted to an engaged, knocked-up woman when there are so many unattached, non-pregnant, younger women out there dying to meet a single, employed male. Or is there?

"Hey, you know that new intern everyone keeps talking about at your work?"

"Yeah. What about her?" I asked hesitantly.

"I met her last night, after you went home." I didn't *go* home. They're the ones who *dropped me off* at home.

"You did? What's she like?"

"Well, I didn't think she was all that much. But Charlie could not stop staring at her, and she was loving it. He even bought her a drink, the asshole."

"Is she skinny?"

"Yep. But, worse even, she seems nice."

"Fuck."

"Yeah, I know. I'm going to make sure Charlie stays far away from her. You better watch it. She might be on the make for my man, but she's definitely on the make for a full-time job. A man is always easier to replace than a job."

"Oh, I'm not worried," I tell Heather.

"I would be. Once you go on maternity leave, she can really make her mark."

God.

I e-mail Seth back saying he's on for Sunday night. Sunday night does not a date make. And he does know that I'm pregnant and that I have a fiancé. I'm going to a movie with Cute Single Man, if only to prove to Heather (and Sexy Young Intern) that I am still an attractive, sought-after woman, just like them. Except for the fact that my pants are a little tighter and that I'll be drinking Perrier instead of Pinot Noir for a few more months, *nothing* is going to change just because I'm knocked up. Absolutely nothing. You can quote me on that.

THE SECOND TRIMESTER

a.k.a. The Fat Months

APRIL 21

Nothing *is* going to change, I swear, except I now have to fit things like obstetrician and ultrasound appointments into my schedule, as opposed to— make that, as well as—manicure and facial appointments. Where, oh where, do women find the time to have a full-time job, be pregnant, have a baby, and, all the while, worry about bikini and underarm waxes? After I have had an ultrasound and met my obstetrician, so he can tell me everything looks as it should, I figure I can tell everyone—the rest of my family, friends who don't know already, my boss—The Big News.

Nothing *is* going to change, except I found myself this morning—a Monday morning, to add to the pain—out and about at the crack of dawn.

I usually don't schedule appointments before 11 a.m. because (a) I know I will sleep through them and (b) I know I will sleep through them. I needn't have worried. I couldn't fall asleep last night anyway, for fear I would sleep through my alarm and get off on the wrong foot with my obstetrician, who would think I was flaky and irresponsible for missing my first ever baby appointment. I couldn't have him thinking that I was irresponsible—at least, I couldn't have him thinking that I was irresponsible before he even met me. Trying to fall asleep was like trying to fall asleep before a final exam. I was more worried about missing the appointment than I was about the appointment itself. Plus I had worked harder than I have ever worked at anything to get in to see the doctor in the first place.

The process was more frustrating than getting an appointment at a trendy hair salon. At least at the most popular hair salon in town, someone always picks up the phone during business hours to tell you snottily, "Good luck! Roberto doesn't have any openings until the New Year. But we can put you on a waiting list if you'd like, in case we have a cancellation." But the doctor's receptionist never even picked up the phone—not during business hours or after hours or before office hours. And she certainly didn't return any calls either. The first five times I called Dr. G.'s office, over a two-week period at varying times throughout the day and night, it went straight into voice mail.

Once the recorded voice mail message even had the nerve to tell me, "This mailbox is full. Please try again later," making me wonder exactly how many pregnant women were out there leaving desperate messages for their obstetricians.

"Ronnie! No one at Dr. G.'s office will call me back. I've left five messages in ten days. Why don't they like me? Do you think they don't like me?"

"They're impossible to get a hold of," Ronnie acknowledged. "You basically have to be in tears for them to get back to you. Tears usually work, so don't be afraid to turn on the waterworks."

I had decided not to do any research about obstetricians in town, just as I had decided not to read about anything to do with pregnancy. Why would I when I had Ronnie, my most neurotic, most obsessive mother friend? She talks to at least one doctor a day about something. If she wakes up with a headache, she's convinced she has a brain tumor. If one of her kids has a mosquito bite, she assumes they're going to get West Nile virus. If Ronnie thought Dr. G. was good enough to deliver her three children, then he was good enough for me. And compared to Ronnie, I would look like a sane and easygoing patient. Ronnie, after all, is the Cher of all mothers. She's a diva.

I tried Dr. G.'s office again. It became sort of a game in a "You're not calling me back? Well I'm not going to stop calling you then" kind of way, much like when I need to interview celebrities for the paper and their publicity representatives don't return my calls. I keep calling and calling until they do, even if it is just to get me off their backs. I was not going to lose this game of Getting a Hold of the Obstetrician. I can be stubborn. I'm a Taurus.

Someone, finally, picked up! I was so shocked to hear a human voice at the other end of the line, I almost forgot whom and why I was calling.

"Yes, this is Rebecca Eckler. Finally, you picked up! I've left half a dozen messages for you already," I huffed to the faceless voice.

There was no response. It was like this woman hadn't listened to any of my messages, ever.

"I really would like Dr. G. to be my obstetrician. I hear he's the best. But I'm getting worried because I'm almost at three months and nobody has called me back," I continued. "I'm getting really nervous. Should I find someone else?" I heard my voice crack. I didn't have to pretend I was going to cry. I was so frustrated by that point, the tears were on the verge of coming anyway. But whether it was the "Should I find someone else?" line or the flattering "I hear he's the best" line, something clicked. She booked me an appointment.

Ronnie had also warned me to grab the earliest appointment available in the day, "or else you will be waiting for hours."

"Can I get an early-morning appointment?" I asked.

Which is how I found myself at an ultrasound clinic at 7:45 a.m. After the ultrasound, I was to go straight to Dr. G.'s office, which was a five-minute walk away, to meet him.

"And write down every single question you can think of," Ronnie advised. "Because this is your chance to get all your worries out in one go. You already know how impossible it is to get a hold of him. And I'm sure you have a million questions for him."

"Right. Yes, of course I do. I'll bring a notepad. I'll probably fill it up, I'll have so many questions by then."

I was shocked when I walked into the ultrasound clinic. There were already five women, in varying degrees of largeness, waiting. Ronnie was right. By noon, I imagined, this place would be as busy as a Kate Spade sample sale a week before Christmas.

Immediately, the one thing I noticed all these women had in common, aside from being pregnant, was a man sitting beside them. I hadn't felt bad before about not having the fiancé at my side, but now I felt a little jolt. Where were all the single mothers I keep hearing about? Perhaps I should have rented a man for a couple of hours. I knew Cute Single Man would have come along if I'd asked him. Though, really, all the men in the waiting area *did* look bored. Waiting in any doctor's office is always boring, unless the *National Enquirer* is on hand, which it wasn't. I won't demand that the fiancé come with me to any of these appointments. What's the point? It's not like he has to be there. It's not like he has the uterus.

Still, I felt underdressed without a man accessory at my side. It was like going out without a purse, or forgetting to put on your engagement ring. Something felt missing.

After twenty minutes of waiting, asking myself if all the other couples were pitying me or wondering why I was all alone, I was called in.

So far in this pregnancy, I've felt like I'm the first woman to ever get pregnant. But I realized immediately that I was nothing special to the ultrasound technician, who barely managed to grunt out a "hello" when she led me into the room. She didn't even offer up her name.

She told me to lie down on the bed, pull up my shirt, and lower my pants. (There's a reason your mother always told you to wear clean underwear to the doctor. Note to self: At least wear a pair of underwear next time.) The technician squeezed some stuff on my stomach—yuck—and started rubbing an instrument over my belly while watching a 1985-style computer monitor I couldn't see from where I was lying.

"Does everything look okay?" I asked the second she began whatever it was she was doing.

"Hmmm," came the response.

Three minutes later I tried again.

"Does everything look okay?"

"Hmmm." Something must be wrong! Something must be wrong! Why wasn't she answering me?

"Can I see what you're looking at?" I asked.

"Hmmm. In a minute," she mumbled.

She worked away for ten minutes in silence, and then I couldn't stand it any longer.

"Does. Everything. Look. Okay?" I asked her—again—tersely.

"I'm not a doctor. You'll have to talk to your doctor."

Crap. Didn't she understand what I was going through?

"Here's your baby's head," she finally said, in a monotone, turning the monitor so I could see what she had been looking at. "And that's the heartbeat."

"Oh my God! That's so amazing. There's actually something growing in me," I screeched. "Isn't that amazing? It looks so weird. Doesn't it look weird?" The thing growing in me looked, in fact, like an actual baby, albeit a bony, skeletal baby with a head the size of a watermelon. But the form was there.

"Hmmm," came the response. I think she could have at least attempted to smile at my awe. That would have been a nice thing to do. I mean, really, how hard is it to fake a smile? Had this woman never been to a cocktail party?

I wanted a souvenir to take with me. What's the point of having an ultrasound if you can't carry a picture of it around with you at all times to annoy your friends and family?

She printed off two photos and handed them to me. "Go to the front desk with these. You have to pay $10 for them. We'll send copies over to your obstetrician now."

Gaaa! I had to pay for them? Shouldn't the photos have been free—a perk for being pregnant? (Note to self: Next time you go for an ultrasound, wear underwear *and* bring your wallet.) I did what any other expectant mother would do upon being handed pictures of her child for the first time and knowing she didn't have any money in her purse: I shoved them in my bag and ran like the wind, not looking back for fear that someone in a white coat would be chasing after me. Make no mistake, I don't think stealing is right. I will not raise my child to be a thief. But it was a picture of *my* baby in *my* stomach. I deserve it. Especially after everything I've been through.

I called the fiancé from my cellphone after leaving the clinic. He wasn't picking up—he was probably still asleep like everyone else not getting ultrasounds—so I left a message. "I just saw our child for the first time at the ultrasound appointment. It seems to have an extremely large alien-like head, just like you! Going to the obstetrician now. Call me back."

The fiancé called while I was in Dr. G.'s waiting room. I had been trying to think of questions to ask Dr. G., just like Ronnie told me. On the back of a receipt I found in my bag, I had written down "So how much weight will I gain?" and "How long will it take to lose the weight after?" and "Any suggestions on how to tell my boss?" and "Do you think that Sexy Young Intern will get my job?" and "Do you think the baby so far is cute?" But I had scratched all of those out. I'm sure those weren't the type of questions I was supposed to be asking my obstetrician. A shrink or a good friend, maybe, but not a baby doctor.

"You didn't tell me you were going to get an ultrasound or that you had a doctor's appointment," the fiancé said.

"Yes I did."

"No, no you didn't."

"I didn't?"

"No, you didn't."

"Really? I think I must have."

"No, you think wrong. You never told me."

"I didn't? Are you sure?"

"Yes! Don't you think I'd remember something like that?"

I'm not sure how that happened. It's true, I'm sure the fiancé would have remembered my telling him something like that. Perhaps I didn't think he was used to the idea of me being pregnant yet and I didn't want to bore him with every little detail about the pregnancy. Perhaps I thought he wouldn't care. Or, most likely, I just totally forgot to mention it. I am pregnant. I do have Baby Brain. I'm amazed I can even remember my name.

"Oh . . . anyway, I saw the baby alien thing growing in me. I saw the head! It's so freaky weird. And I heard the heartbeat. It was beating so fast. But she/he is really, really cute."

"So I guess you really are pregnant then?" the fiancé asked.

"Um, duh, yes. And I have pictures. Oh . . . they just called me in to see Dr. G. I gotta run."

"Wait. Who is Dr. G.?"

"He's my obstetrician. I told you about him. I must have. He was Ronnie's obstetrician."

"You didn't tell me that!"

"Yes I did."

"No you didn't."

"Really?"

"Really."

"I promise to call you right after."

"Beck?"

"Yes?"

"Don't forget, okay?"

"Right."

Dr. G. is a very nice man. He reminds me of my grandfather, balding and soft-spoken, except he wears scrubs. My grandfather has never worn scrubs. First I had to get blood taken, a process which is never fun. I also had to pee, on demand, on a stick, which was okay because I always have to pee these days. Unfortunately, after I finished peeing on the stick, I dropped it on the washroom floor. What was I to do? I couldn't pee again. I had used up all my pee. So I gave it to one of the nurses anyway, praying that Clorox, or whatever they use to clean the washroom floors, wouldn't ruin the test.

Dr. G. asked me a bunch of questions about my

health and the health of my family. And, of course, he asked me the First Day of my Last Period. After I told him, he told me that my due date would be October 20.

"But let's say October 22nd. Because that's my birthday," Dr. G. said.

Oh. Apparently, due dates really aren't that scientific.

I admitted to him, much to my embarrassment, that I was a smoker. I figured that he would yell at me about how bad it is for the child, about how it was a matter of life and death, and that hearing him insist that I stop smoking immediately would finally force me to quit once and for all. But that didn't exactly happen.

"Well, my mother was a smoker when she was pregnant with me. And I was a smoker for many years. I know how hard it is to quit. I understand that it really is an addiction. You should definitely cut back, though, and keep me posted on your progress. Whatever you do, do *not* tell anyone else that you are a smoker because they will lecture you," Dr. G. said.

Eeek! I had needed him—a doctor—to tell me I was an evil, evil woman who was weak for being a smoker in the first place. I *wanted* him to lecture me.

"I know. I know. It's so bad for the baby, right?" I asked, pressing him. "Right?"

"There are studies that show smokers have babies with slightly lower birth weights," he said. "I don't need to lecture you on smoking, though."

Yes, yes, you do! Especially because I *would* rather have a seven-pound baby come out from Down There than a ten-pound baby, so the lower-birth-weight argument doesn't really convince me that smoking is such an awful thing.

"Do you have any questions for me?"

"Yes. Do you think it's weird that a Cute Single Man asked me to a movie and I went with him last night and I think he has a crush on me but how could he seeing how I'm pregnant and engaged to another man?" I asked. Actually, I didn't say that at all. Though that was on my mind.

What I actually said was "Uh, not really." The truth was I couldn't think of any medical questions to ask him. My scrap paper was blank. Shouldn't I have a million questions?

"Let's get you weighed then. What's your normal weight?"

"About a hundred pounds. Sometimes a little less, depending on whether I'm having a bloated day or not. You know, salt and all."

I stood on the scale (first taking off my shoes, of course) and held my breath. I knew I had already gained some weight. My pants are tighter around the waist than they used to be. Some of them don't even button up. I wear long shirts over the pants that don't button up (shhh!), and sometimes I can feel my thighs rub together when I'm walking and wearing skirts, which, trust me, was traumatic when I first noticed. Not as traumatic as what happened next, though.

"You are now 114 pounds."

"I've gained fourteen pounds in three months! *I've gained fourteen pounds in three months?* I'VE GAINED FOURTEEN POUNDS IN THREE MONTHS? Is that normal? *Is that normal?* IS THAT NORMAL?"

"Yes, that's fine. We don't worry about small women like you gaining weight. It's good to gain weight. I'm not worried."

Well, that makes one of us. I am worried. I am very, very worried.

Suddenly the elation I had felt at first seeing the alien-looking baby with the watermelon-size head growing in my stomach was gone. I couldn't believe I'd gained that much weight so quickly. I have never weighed that much before, not even during freshman year at university when all I ate was Kraft Dinner. I have never weighed that much before, not even when everything in my life was going perfectly.

I tried to perk up when I called the fiancé.

"Okay, we're good to go," I told him. "The doctor says everything looks good. We can tell everyone now. But there is one thing . . ."

"But what? What's wrong? You're not having twins, are you? Please tell me you're not having twins."

"No, I'm not having twins! It's nothing. It's just that I . . ."

"What? Tell me."

"Well, I've gained fourteen pounds!"

"Is that bad?"

"Well, the doctor says it's fine."

"Beck, you are pregnant, you know."

"Yeah, yeah, I know. You're right. We should look into obstetricians where you are, too. In case we decide I'll have the baby there."

I hadn't told Dr. G. that I'm not 100 percent certain I'm going to have him deliver the baby. The fiancé and I haven't decided for sure where I will give birth. We still have time to work out the details. I was just relieved that, so far, aside from the fourteen-pound weight gain, everything looks fine. I decided to celebrate my first ultrasound by treating myself to a Big Mac and super-sized fries. What's a couple more thousand calories anyway? It would be my last trip to McDonald's.

Noon

Back at my apartment, four and a half hours and one Big Mac after I left to go to the appointment, it's time to tell the boss. What's the proper etiquette for telling your boss you're going to have a baby? One of my colleagues, I remember, didn't tell the boss she was pregnant until two weeks before she was set to give birth. She continued going into the office and wore really baggy sweaters to camouflage the growing bump. She got away with it. She told me afterward she just assumed everyone thought she had gained a lot of weight but were too polite to say anything.

God, this is going to be hard. I don't want the

boss to take me less seriously or to think that I'm not committed to my job. But I have to tell him. I don't want people to think I'm just getting fat. I could call him, but that would be weird, considering I've never called my boss at the office before and don't know his direct number. Should I set up a meeting with him? That, too, would be weird. The only time I've set up meetings with him is when I've wanted a raise. If I call to ask for a meeting, he'll probably think I am going to ask for another raise and then he'll never return my phone call. Or maybe he'll think someone in my family has died. I don't want to turn the fact that I am pregnant into something so serious and somber. This is, after all, supposed to be good news, or at least a pleasant surprise. That's what I want him to think, at least.

I decide to go the e-mail route. E-mail has become a girl's best friend and her worst enemy. It's made dumping men easier. It's made men dumping us easier, too. It's made canceling plans easier for everyone. And now e-mail has, apparently, made telling your boss you are pregnant easier, too. Plus you can write drafts of the letter before you hit Send and your whole life changes in one nanosecond.

Subject: I'm pregnant!!!
Message: I'm pregnant. Just thought you should know sooner than later. Not because you're the father. So don't you go worrying about that! Ha ha . . .

No, that won't work. It's too flippant. It's in bad taste. I don't want him to think I'm crazy and planning to sue him for sexual harassment or something.

Subject: Well, it's finally happened . . .
Message: I'm three months pregnant. I am woman. Hear me roar!

No, no, no. What am I thinking?

Subject: I have something to tell you.
Message: The fiancé and I got drunk three months ago and didn't use protection, and now I'm with child . . .

ARGH!

Subject: Don't hate me because I'm fat . . .
Message: No need to hire anyone to take my job just because I'm about to get bigger, maybe even fat. A.k.a. pregnant. Don't worry. I'll still be the same hard-working employee I have always been and will continue to be the best person for the job. I promise. I promise. I promise. So no need to find a replacement or, let's say, hire that younger intern to take over my position.

ARGH! ARGH! ARGH!

Okay, it's clear there's no good way of doing this other than to do it. Here goes . . .

Subject: Important News!
Message: The fiancé and I are three months pregnant. Well, I am three months pregnant. I'm very happy about it. I would like to write about it for tomorrow's paper. There is some funny stuff related to finding out. I think readers will be very entertained. Will be well read.

I figure I could at least show the boss, while in the process of telling him I am pregnant, that I am still going to work hard, that I still care about the newspaper.

Less than five minutes later, my computer blings.

Subject: Re: Important News!
Message: Congratulations. That is exciting news. Will you be taking maternity leave? And, yes, please write about it for tomorrow's paper. I'm sure it will be great.

Phew. That wasn't too awful. In fact, it really was anticlimactic. Didn't he care? I must learn to not overanalyze. I really haven't thought about maternity leave, though, I mean, I've thought about it in that I think a year off would be really nice, like an extended paid vacation where you can throw your baby on your back with one of those funky baby-knapsack-thingies and tour Europe. Though maybe I'm not the type of woman who can take off from work for so long without wanting to get back into the "game." I hear about women all the time who go back to work three weeks after giving birth because they are so worried they are going to lose the position they worked so hard to get in the first place. I do love my job. Will I love watching a baby more? Somehow I can't imagine changing diapers as being more enjoyable than getting paid to interview celebrities and attend fabulous bar openings. But maybe I can be that type of woman?

I call to warn the fiancé he'd better tell everyone he knows or who needs to know about me being pregnant because I'm writing about it in tomorrow's paper. Then I get down to work, keeping the ultrasound photo next to my computer for inspiration. The alien child is so damn cute I can't keep my eyes off of it. How will that watermelon-size head come out from Down There? I won't worry about that now. I have to work.

5:30 p.m.

Bling! My e-mail goes off. I just sent my pregnancy story in ten minutes ago. Oh. My. God. The e-mail is from Sexy Young Intern.

Subject: Your Big Surprise!
Message: Congratulations. I can't believe you are pregnant! Everyone in the office is talking about it. Word travels fast here. Will you be moving to be with the fiancé now? Any cravings? Are you going to leave work?

Argh! What a bitch! She probably wants me to be craving ice cream so I'll get fat. She's probably already plotting to get my job, sucking up to the boss right this second. This isn't going to be good. I delete the e-mail without responding. I'll blame it on my pregnancy hormones if I run into her and she asks why I never wrote back.

APRIL 22

Gaaa!! The story of my pregnancy made it to the front page of the newspaper. "REBECCA ECKLER IS PREGNANT!" it screamed along the top of the front page. Now everyone will know. I turned on my computer to see hundreds of e-mails with the subject heading "Congratulations" waiting for me in my Inbox. It was overwhelming. Who knew that so many people—including readers I've never met—could be happy for me? I wasn't used to it. I couldn't deal with it.

The fiancé called.

"I'm so annoyed."

"What? What? You didn't like the story. What's wrong with it?"

"No, the story was fine. But people have been calling me all morning. I can't get any work done."

"I know. I know. Me neither!"

"If I hear one more time how having a baby 'changes everything' but that it's 'so rewarding' and that 'it's the best thing I'll ever do,' I'm going to hurt someone."

It's true. Almost every e-mail and phone call

I've received says the same thing. "It's the most rewarding thing you'll ever do" and "It changes everything. Just you wait and see" and "All your priorities will change" and "Enjoy every minute of the pregnancy, because after the baby is born you will never have a quiet moment again." And shut up, shut up, shut up.

The fiancé and I are cynics. We don't like to be told how rewarding anything is. We don't like to be told to enjoy anything. Neither of us deals well with change, either.

"I'm going to turn off my phone," the fiancé said.

"Me too. But don't be too annoyed. Just think how rewarding this will all be. Ha ha."

"Goodbye, Beck."

Still, aside from being annoyed by everyone telling me how "everything changes," I can't help but gloat. My newspaper is really selling the story that I am pregnant. Maybe this won't be so bad for my career. Maybe I can still be fabulous, albeit fabulously pregnant. Who isn't interested, for example, in designer diaper bags and designer baby clothes? Could being pregnant possibly be good for my career? Take that, Sexy Young Intern! I am pregnant and you are not. Maybe I'll end up on the pages of *Us Weekly*, under the heading "Celebrity Parents and Their Tots." Isn't that every woman's dream?

It's amazing—I no longer have morning sickness. I woke up and felt fine. How did that happen? People had told me the morning sickness would go away after the first three months, and it did, almost exactly three months to the day. Amazing.

It's a good thing too, because I have a very big day planned. I've been putting off doing this for three months, but it can't wait any longer. It has to be done today unless I plan never to leave my house again. I have to go bra shopping.

I realized the importance of this yesterday, when the one remaining bra that kind of fit snapped open as I bent down. Yes, it happened: my pregnant breasts broke my bra. Plus, panty lines are bad, but bra lines are hideous. I've decided to walk to my neighborhood lingerie shop, where they know me and where I feel comfortable having the salesgirls feel me up as they take measurements.

"Well, you haven't been in here for a while," Jen, the friendly salesgirl, said when I walked in. "What's new?"

"Um, well, I'm pregnant. And my breasts are huge now. I need new bras."

Jen looked at me, wide-eyed, as if she had just seen a rat running through her store, but she didn't say anything.

"Well, you can wipe that shocked look off your face now," I told her.

"I'm sorry. I just—well, wow, you're pregnant? I'm stunned."

"Yeah, me too. But let's try to get over our shock, shall we? I desperately need new bras."

"Okay, let's get you measured." Jen measured me. "Okay, wow, you're now a double-D."

"Double-D? What was I before? Oh, and, once again, you can wipe that shocked look off your face."

"I think you were a B. I can't believe you are still wearing that bra. You must be so uncomfortable."

"Yep."

"Let me grab you a few bras to try on. I'll be right back. Wow . . . double-D," she said again, shaking her head in disbelief.

"Okay, but make sure they have underwire. I think I need the support more than ever now. Plus, I like underwire. It's sexier," I told her.

"Well, you really shouldn't be wearing under-wire bras now, you know. Your breasts need to move around when you're pregnant."

What? No sushi? No alcohol? No medicine? No Diet Coke? No cigarettes? And now no underwire? Does it never end?

"Listen, Jen. I really want bras with underwire. I promise to come back in a couple months and get some without. But, for now, let's stick to underwire."

"Oh, you'll be back. Probably in a few weeks. Your breasts are going to continue to grow, you know."

They can't possibly! If my breasts get any bigger, I'm going to need some sort of apparatus to hold me upright.

Jen walked off.

"Here you go. I grabbed you a couple with underwire and another kind I just want you to try on. Trust me."

I couldn't believe what Jen had handed me. They weren't bras. They were tablecloths.

"Oh my God. Those are so unsexy!" I cried to her. "And what's with this white one? What is that?"

"Just try it on. Please? For me."

First I tried on two black double-D bras—with underwire—and one purple lacy one. Despite the sexy colors, they looked like bras someone's grandmother would wear.

Then I tried on the white bra. It was 100 percent cotton and had huge, thick straps the width of my hand. It was possibly the ugliest bra I have ever seen. Whoever made this bra definitely wasn't trying to impress a new lover.

It was . . . heaven. Jen came into the changing room to check on me.

"This bra is the most comfortable thing ever. It's like I'm wearing nothing. I'll take it. But what is this plastic clip here, right over the cup?"

"Oh, it's a nursing bra. I didn't want to tell you. Just unhook the clip and you can breastfeed. See? It's practical as well as comfortable," she laughed.

"I can't believe I'm buying a nursing bra and I'm not even four months pregnant! This is all so sad."

But I wore the bra out of the store. I will have to remember to hide it, or take it off, when I see the fiancé. It really is that unattractive. It will scare him. It isn't a bra so much as a parachute or something.

APRIL 25

The fiancé called.

"Boy, you're in trouble."

"What? What did I do?" Did the fiancé know about Sunday's movie night with Cute Single Man? I'm still feeling guilty about it. We had seen a seven o'clock show (a late show seemed too much like a date), but after, because it was still early, it had seemed wrong to end the night. I invited him back to my place, where I handed him a beer and poured myself a glass of water.

The initial reason for agreeing to go to a movie with Cute Single Man was to prove to Heather that a guy could be attracted to me even though I am pregnant. And Cute Single Man does seem to like me, and I'm not convinced he likes me just as a "friend." After all, we both already have friends and I'm not that interesting.

"You know," Cute Single Man said to me, checking out my apartment, "you should really put a piece of wood or a bar along your sliding glass door. You're on the ground floor. Someone could easily break in." It was kind of nice to have someone be so concerned about my security. I hate to admit it, but I had fun with Cute Single Man. I felt, well, single, out on a first date. Nothing happened. In fact, I've made a promise to myself never to see him again, though he did make me laugh. It just seemed wrong. I haven't told the fiancé about it, because how would I explain it all? Somehow I don't think "Well, Heather made me feel ugly and bad and I needed to feel better about being pregnant" was going to cut it.

"Yes, you're in trouble," the fiancé repeated.

"Um, what did I do?" Was it possible that one of the fiancé's friends saw us at the movies and ratted on me?

"Well, Jason just called me." Phew. Jason lives in the same building as the fiancé. There's no way he could have seen me out at the movies with a man who isn't the father of my child.

"So what?" I asked.

"His girlfriend is now all over him to get pregnant because you are."

"Really? I thought Jason was the one who laughed at you when you told him I was pregnant."

"He did! That was a wonderful response. Anyway, they got into a huge fight about it and she demanded to know if they were ever going to have a baby together. I think they figure if we're doing it, then everybody must be doing it."

"Yikes."

Women are like this, I told the fiancé. I wasn't surprised. If all our friends are single, we want to be single. If the most unexpected people—like the fiancé and I—are pregnant, they think it's time for them to be pregnant too. If we could do it, after all, then *anyone* could.

Maybe everyone *is* pregnant. I decided to go back to the gym today. It's been way too long, and now that my morning sickness is over there's really no good excuse not to go. Plus I don't want my butt getting any bigger. I decided to make plans to meet my gym friend Sara there, so we could take a spin class together and then go for eggs. I am so happy I went. Guess what? Sara is pregnant! After our spin class—which proved to be a tad more difficult to get through because every time I bent over on the bike I got the urge to pee—we were looking over the gym class schedule while talking to one of the instructors.

"You shouldn't take the FITT class anymore," the instructor told me. "There's a lot of jumping around and your heartbeat shouldn't go faster than 140 when you're pregnant. But Sara, do you want to sign up for it?"

"Um, well, I can't," Sara said hesitantly, pointing at me. "Same as her."

"What?" the instructor and I said in unison, looking at Sara.

"I'm pregnant too. Two months," she said.

"Yah!" I screamed, giving her a hug. Trust me, if any of my friends told me they were pregnant before I knew I was pregnant, they would most likely have got a stunned silence out of me and maybe a "Way to go." But now I need as many friends as possible to go through this non-drinking, non-smoking, going-to-bed-early experience with me.

Over brunch, I got the details. Sara is a couple of years older than me, has been married for three years, and recently started a new job as a publicist for a record company. I knew she wanted to get pregnant one day—that was never a question—but not three months after she got a new job.

"We decided I'd go off the pill a couple months ago. But then I got this job and we thought we'd put trying on hold for a while. I didn't want my work thinking I took the job only for the maternity benefits—which are, I'll admit, better than the benefits at my old job. Anyway, he came in me only once. I thought the pill would still be in my system. They say it can take a year to stop working and I've been on the pill for fifteen years. But all it took was that one time."

"I know. One time is all it takes! Amazing, isn't it?"

"Um, Beck."

"Yeah?"

"You have, um, eggs Benedict all over you."

I looked down at my shirt. There was egg dribble all over my breasts, and breadcrumbs down my new deep cleavage.

"Oh God. I'm not used to my new breasts being there yet. I spill everything on me now. Just you wait," I said, mortified, trying to wipe out the crumbs that were down my bra.

"I can't wait to get the breasts! I'm so excited about that."

"Well, you won't be too excited when it's hot outside and you notice you're sweating in your cleavage. It's quite nasty. Also, I find myself opening doors and hitting myself in the stomach with the door now. I'm not used to my new stomach either. Anyway, how excited is your husband about all of this?"

"He's so excited. He won't let me smoke anymore and he even smokes his nightly joint outside the house now. Isn't that nice?"

It's amazing the things husbands will do for their pregnant wives.

APRIL 30

My thirtieth birthday is May 11, less than two weeks away. The fiancé has decided to come to town and throw a dinner party at a chic restaurant for me and thirty of my friends. Because my birthday falls on Mother's Day this year—what are the chances?— I asked him if I will be getting two presents, one for my birthday and one for Mother's Day. It made sense to me, what with me carrying his child and all.

"No. You're not a mother yet," he answered.

"But I am. Kind of. I'm pregnant. There's an actual living thing growing in me. I'm supposed to be taking care of it, so I'm already kind of a mother."

"I have to actually see the child before I will consider you a mother. And are you really taking care of it? Have you quit smoking?"

"Well, I'm down to one a week."

"Are you lying to me?"

"Yes. But I am down to one a day. That's pretty good."

"Are you still lying to me?"

"Yes, but I'm down to three a day. That's better, isn't it?"

"Yes, that's great."

"So do I get two presents?"

"Do I get a Father's Day present in June?"

"No. What have you done really? Except come in me? And in October, I'm giving you the most rewarding gift ever, as some have told you."

"Well, if I don't get a Father's Day gift, then you don't get a Mother's Day gift."

"Fine. It's not fair, though."

It hit me that this would be my last Mother's Day ever as a non-mother. Well, at least next year I will get a Mother's Day gift. But I think I'll start saving the "I'm giving you the most rewarding gift ever" line for when there's something really big that I really, really want. It's too good to use liberally.

I think I may have started a trend. Joanne, a trainer at the gym, told me today that she is pregnant too. Maybe pregnancy is contagious. Joanne's pregnancy announcement made me feel especially happy because Joanne is definitely a downtown "cool" type of girl. She has an eyebrow piercing and changes her hair color as often as most people change their bedsheets. Today her hair was blue. She, too, is not married to her boyfriend, but they live together. If a blue-haired, eyebrow-pierced gym trainer is ecstatic about being pregnant, I can be too.

"So, are you still working out as much?" I asked her.

"Not as hard as I used to," she told me. "I just listen to my body. You have to listen to your body and it will tell you when enough is enough."

Huh? I hate when people say, "Just listen to your body." What does that even mean? My body hasn't been telling me anything, except to eat french fries every day. I have listened. I've eaten french fries every single day of my pregnancy so far.

"Do you have any cravings yet?" Joanne asked me.

"No, not really. Just french fries, I guess, and Big Macs. But I've always loved french fries. You?"

"Just mangoes."

It just figures that the pregnant gym trainer would crave something healthy. It's enough to drive an inherently lazy girl to super-sized fries to make herself feel better.

MAY 4

I'm starting to worry about not having abnormal cravings. I knew one pregnant woman who craved the smell of gasoline so badly during her pregnancy that she forced her husband to take her for drives to the gas station every night. I'm not sure how healthy that craving would be. Maybe it's best that I'm not craving anything interesting.

MAY 5

11:00 a.m.

If I don't get a Starbucks iced latte in the next five minutes, I. Will. Kill. Somebody. I will actually physically hurt whoever gets in the way of me and my iced latte.

11:25 a.m.

This decaf iced latte is the best thing I have ever tasted. I've never had one before, either. Interesting. Hey! The cravings are here! Yippee! The cravings are here!

4:00 p.m.

Cute Single Man called. "Do you want to go to a movie tonight?" he asked. "There are so many movies I want to see. And I got you a little something."

"You did?"

"Yes. I think you'll like it."

Do I dare go out with him again? What else do I have to do? Shannon, Lena, and Heather haven't called me all weekend, though I really hadn't noticed until now. Why haven't they called? What are they doing without me?

"Um, well. Okay, I guess I could see an early movie," I told him. Why not? It's not so wrong, is it?

"How's the baby?"

"Um, good. Everything seems to be good."

"Should I pick you up at seven?"

"Yeah, okay."

"Hey, I've kind of missed you." Gaa! How to respond? How to respond?

"See you at seven," I said, before hanging up. He misses me? He has a present for me? And he asked how the baby was? Either Cute Single Man is the best friend out there for a pregnant woman or this is going to lead to nothing but disaster. What the hell. It's just a movie. And maybe we could stop for an iced latte along the way. I'd have to go out later and get one anyway.

Cute Single Man bought me a padlock for my back gate and a bar for my sliding glass door. I like Cute Single Man. Not in that way. But at least he seems to care. I can't go out with him anymore, though. I love my fiancé and called to tell him so, right after Cute Single Man dropped me off from the movie. Okay, we also went for an iced latte. That was imperative.

"Hey, it's me."

"What are you doing?" the fiancé asked.

"Nothing. I went to a movie."

"With who?"

"Lena. Hey, how come you never ask me how I'm feeling? It's the least you can do. I am pregnant. Don't you worry about me at all?"

"Beck, what's going on?" Truth is, I had no idea where that came from. It just came out. I was angry at the fiancé for seeming not to care as much as Cute Single Man, though I know he cares more. Goddamn these hormones. It must be the hormones.

"Beck, I never ask you how you are feeling because you tell me how you're feeling before I have the chance to ask."

"Yeah. That's true."

"But I promise to ask more often from now on, okay?"

"Okay. That's all I'm asking."

Today, when I was rummaging through my washroom cupboard looking for some conditioner, an
o.b. tampon fell to the floor and rolled toward the
bathtub. That's weird, I thought to myself. Just
seeing the tampon made me pause for a moment.
It's strange not getting your period for so long. It's
funny how you can forget about something that
basically has ruined your life each month for fifteen years. Seeing the tampon was like having a
former high school boyfriend's phone number
pop into your head out of the blue ten years after
you've broken up. It makes you pause—WHOA!—
and question where the heck it came from and how
you could have forgotten the number you once
knew by heart in the first place.

MAY 9

The fiancé is arriving tonight and has rented the
top floor of a restaurant for my birthday party
tomorrow. All my friends are coming—Dana,
Heather and her boyfriend, Shannon and the guy
she's seeing, Lena, Ronnie and her husband,
pregnant Vivian and her husband, pregnant Sara
and her husband, and a few of my colleagues from
work—along with a handful of the fiancé's friends.
It should be a great night, a good mix of singles
and pregnant women. I'm trying to bring every-

one closer—like the United Nations—to prove that we pregnant women aren't so different. No, I'm not really. But it sounds good. In fact, tomorrow night will be the first night I've been in the company of so many pregnant women.

Dana and I made plans to go shopping this afternoon. She absolutely needs a new outfit to wear to the party. Our shopping excursion didn't last long. It was too depressing. I'm at the stage where some of my pre-pregnancy clothes still fit, and I don't want to waste money on clothes that will fit for only another two weeks. I'm not exactly sure what is going to happen to my body. I do know that I will never buy maternity clothes. When I get bigger, I plan to buy normal clothes, in larger sizes. I'm going to remain a funky dresser, and I probably won't need to go bigger than a size 12.

"I've only been to the gym five times this week," Dana moaned to me as we were walking along the street. "I feel disgusting and fat."

"I can't have this conversation," I told her. "I've been to the gym about two times in three months! You're going to have to shut up with your moaning about only going to the gym five times in one week." Dana was the one who introduced me to the concept of going to the gym twice a day, which she often does and which I used to do occasionally.

As we entered store after store, it became clear to me that, to the outside world, I don't yet look pregnant. I guess I just look chunkier. Every time I tried something on, the salespeople would be all over me, like ants to crumbs. "That looks great on you," they'd profess. "You should definitely get that."

So I would tell them, "Well, I'm pregnant. Do you think these will fit me in a month?"

"You're pregnant?" they'd respond, surprised. I suppose it should have made me feel content to still be able to pass as a non-pregnant woman. But then I thought, Well if I'm trying this on and they say that it looks great on me and that I don't look pregnant, then what they're really saying is that I look fat, because I know I'm not as skinny as I was. Which is why I didn't end up buying anything. Watching Dana try on skin-tight pants became increasingly annoying.

"Maybe I should get a shirt printed that reads, 'I'm not fat, I'm pregnant,'" I said to Dana, before claiming to need a nap. Pregnancy is a wonderful excuse to get out of situations you no longer want to be in.

MAY 11

The fiancé and I showed up thirty minutes late to my birthday party last night. Emily Post would have rolled over in her grave if she had seen what went down. The fiancé and I were, in fact, the last ones to arrive at the party thrown for *me* by *him*. It wasn't entirely my fault. Whoever came up with "It was the best of times, it was the worst of times" must have been pregnant. I had my first pregnancy-related getting-ready nervous break-down last night. Neither the fiancé nor I saw it coming. One hour before we had to leave, I jumped in the shower. I had made sure I had plenty of time to dry my hair, put on makeup, and get dressed so we would be the first to arrive. Fifteen minutes before we had to leave, however, I was still sitting on my bed, wrapped in a towel, my hair dripping wet, clothes strewn all around me, bawling my eyes out.

I had nothing to wear. I know women use the "I have nothing to wear" line all the time when they have a million outfits in their closets to choose from. This was entirely different. I really *didn't* have anything to wear. Suddenly, as if it had hap-pened overnight, nothing fit.

"What is going on in here?" the fiancé said, entering the bedroom. He had shaved and was dressed and ready to go. "Why are you crying? What's wrong? What's wrong. Tell me." I was cry-ing so hard, I'm sure he thought I had hurt myself or that someone had died. He looked quite fright-ened, the way men look when they don't know how to deal with female emotional crises.

"I, uh, uh, I have, uh, nothing, n-n-nothing t-t-to wear," I managed to get out, gulping for air. "N-n-nothing f-f-fits."

Most of my sexy, tight tank tops and shirts no longer stretched over my breasts. The ones that did no longer covered my entire stomach. My size 6 low-waisted jeans would not fit over my ass any longer. All my dresses were so skin-tight now I couldn't possibly wear them out in public. You could see fat lines.

"Okay. Okay. Please calm down, Beck. Please. Let's figure this out. What about those jeans you wore last night? They looked good."

"Th-th-they're dirty! I've been w-w-wearing th-th-them all week! They're so s-s-s-stretched out, that's w-w-why they probably s-still fit."

"Ah, come on, Beck. No matter what you wear, you'll still be the best-looking girl in the room," said the fiancé, coming to sit beside me and giving me a hug.

"B-b-but it's m-m-my party! I d-d-don't w-w-want to look like sh-shit!"

"Like I said, that's not possible. You could wear sweatpants if you wanted, and I'd still think you were the best-looking woman there."

"Y-you mean th-that?"

"Yes! Now come on. Put on those dirty jeans, and what about that stretchy black halter-top thing? That probably fits. I like that." I hadn't remembered that shirt. The fiancé was right. It was very stretchy. That could work.

Sometimes the fiancé is the only one who can calm me down. Which is why I love him so much. I decided to take his advice on the outfit, slapped on some makeup, and half-blow-dried my hair. We raced for a taxi. Because of my pregnancy-related dressing nervous breakdown, we were already twenty minutes late.

"Are my eyes still red from crying?" I asked him as we raced up the stairs to my party.

"No. You look great. Plus, it's your party and you can cry if you want to."

"Ha ha."

All of our friends were already there.

"Where were you guys?" they screamed out in unison.

"Sorry! It was my fault. Nothing fit me, so I had a crying fit," I said, trying to turn it into a joke. I was embarrassed about the whole incident. No girl, pregnant or not, should ever let any guy know how much thought she puts into getting ready to go out. Preparing to be attractive is so not an attractive ritual.

It was an awesome night. Everyone got drunk, aside from me and the other pregnant women there. (I did have one glass of red wine, which was heaven. I sipped it slowly, as if it were my last meal.) The food was spectacular, and the presents were amazing. It was my best birthday ever.

But I can't go through that kind of pregnancy-related dressing fit again. Mood swings are one thing, but that meltdown was entirely different. The fiancé and I are going shopping today. I'm buying shirts that are super long, and baggy pants with room to grow into. Actually, I'll let him buy them for me. I'll consider that my Mother's Day gift.

MAY 14

Last night Heather called. "You know, we should all go to Italy for a month for a long vacation. Maybe by next year I could save the money."

"That would be fantastic! Wait . . . next year I'll have a child."

"Oh, right. I forgot. But you just reminded me to take my pill."

"Glad I could be of service." Sheesh. Now I'm a reminder to friends to take their birth control?

MAY 17

I'm dreading the weekend ending. I've been working extra hard recently, to prove to everyone that I'm still a good employee and am not slacking off because I'm pregnant. Pregnancy, last I checked, is not a disability. And I can't have Sexy Young Intern outperforming me. Not yet, anyway. No, not ever.

I've noticed when I go into the office to pick up my mail that many of my colleagues are treating me differently these days. Some of them, who are still single and whom I considered my friends, haven't yet called or even e-mailed to congratulate me on my pregnancy. What is wrong with them? Have I shocked them into silence? Or can they no longer relate to me now that I've crossed to the "dark side"? Others, who do have children, who

KNOCKED UP

never before seemed interested in getting to know me, now want to talk to me and have e-mailed me advice on doctors and nannies. I asked one of my female colleagues, who is the same age as me and who recently got married, if she planned on having children anytime soon. "Oh, my in-laws are totally on our backs to get going on the children thing. But I want to enjoy life a bit more," she told me. "There is plenty of time for children." Ouch! Guess we won't be joining the same mommies' group anytime soon.

I've been writing a ton of pregnancy-related stories recently, including "Talking to Your Stomach," "The Evils of Shopping for Clothes While Pregnant," "Getting a Pregnancy Portrait," and "Why Isn't My Hair Shiny Yet?" I've disappointed some of my readers, who have e-mailed to tell me that my "stuff" is now "boring." Am I? Worse, though, are the readers who write demanding to know when I intend to marry. Apparently they've been talking to my parents. On the other hand, a new audience of modern mothers have sent me their stories of being pregnant, and JPEG photos of their babies. Friends and colleagues, in pregnancy, it seems, come and go. So do readers.

I decided to get takeout sushi tonight. (I know, I know. I'm not supposed to eat sushi. But can I help it if my baby is craving sushi? Plus Ronnie told me I'm allowed to eat cooked sushi, so I ordered shrimp tempura rolls and a cucumber roll, even though all I really wanted was spicy tuna sashimi.) I had my first pregnancy sighting, ironically, in the sushi restaurant as I was waiting for my takeout order to be ready.

"Oh, you're expecting baby!" said the Sushi Man, who knows my face because I'm a regular. I hadn't been there in a couple of months.

"You can tell?" I asked, surprised.

"Oh yes. You pregnant," he said, rubbing his belly in circular motions (at least he didn't rub mine!).

I guess I am showing. I'm showing! I'm showing! I'm showing! Finally, I'm showing!

Oh my God, am I ever showing. On the way back from getting an iced latte this afternoon, I caught the reflection of a pregnant woman in a store window. That woman, it turns out, was me. I was momentarily stunned. I looked almost square, like a big-wheel truck. What happened to my hourglass figure? I used to have hips. I know I used to have hips. I raced home, keeping my eyes firmly glued to the ground. That woman in the reflection couldn't possibly be me. I'm not ready for that woman yet. I won't ever be ready for that woman.

Cute Single Man called me. Somehow, over the past few weeks, we have become—gulp—friends. Tonight we had a nice conversation that lasted about an hour. I told him all about the Sushi Man, who could tell I was pregnant instantly upon seeing me.

"Well, it had to happen," he told me.

"I just don't want to look fat," I said.

"You won't look fat. You'll look pregnant."

We talk almost every day now. He calls under the guise of checking up on me, which is nice. Is he in love with me? Who knows? I do know he doesn't seem to mind when I complain about my fat thighs for twenty minutes. At least he pretends not to mind.

MAY 23

The fiancé had warned me that a package would arrive for me sometime today. He wouldn't tell me what it was, but he did say, "Don't worry if you don't like what's inside. I don't expect you to like it." The package did arrive. It was from my future mother-in-law, one of this child's grandmothers. I ripped it open only to see—GAA! What were those? Maternity clothes? Okay, maybe this wasn't a bad thing. The woman does have good taste. (In the past she has bought me a Prada wallet and makeup case and some funky T-shirts and a Louis Vuitton bag.) There were two pairs of pants and one pair of shorts. What was with those super-thick elastic bands? I don't care what anyone says. Maybe maternity clothes *are* better than they used to be. But slightly better than awful is still awful. I can't wear them. No way. Nuh uh. No chance in hell.

MAY 24

Vivian, our pregnant friend, invited the "girls"—me, Heather, Shannon, and a couple others—over for dinner tonight. She and her husband have just finished redecorating their house, and she wanted to show it off. I was excited, not only to see the house, but because I felt like I hadn't seen Heather and Shannon since my birthday party—and I hadn't. Having another pregnant woman around makes things easier for me too. I don't feel like the odd woman out. Vivian and I could bond over bottled water, I figured, while everyone else got drunk on wine.

I was the first to arrive. "Would you like a glass of wine or champagne?" Vivian asked. "Are you drinking?"

I hadn't had a sip of alcohol since my birthday. I couldn't believe pregnant Vivian was offering me alcohol. Was this a test?

"I'll just stick to water," I said to her. "I'm still eating sushi, drinking coffee and the odd Diet Coke, and smoking the occasional cigarette. The least I can do is not drink alcohol. Are you still drinking?"

"Not really. But I can't say no to a glass of champagne every once in a while. It's my one vice. I do love champagne."

While we were waiting for the others to arrive, I asked for the grand tour. The house was spectacular. The kitchen was fantastic. The guest rooms were charming. The bathrooms were luxurious.

"This is the last room," said Vivian, leading me to a closed door on the second floor. She opened the door and—Gaaa!—there it was, the baby room, all decorated in blue and white. Vivian already knows she's having a boy.

"I can't believe it!" I screeched. "You're having a baby one month ahead of me, which is still another four months away, and you've already done all this? This is amazing." And it was. She had the crib, the change table, and the rocking chair. It was the Baby Room right out of the Pottery Barn catalogue. The crib was made up with sheets, there were stuffed animals everywhere, and a mobile was hung over the crib, ready to be wound up and played. Wait—were those diapers laid out? Vivian, apparently, is the Martha Stewart of pregnant women.

"I'm impressed. I don't even know what a baby room needs aside from a crib," I told her.

Unlike Vivian and her husband, the fiancé and I are both Jewish. We were brought up believing that you shouldn't buy anything for the baby, set anything up for the baby, or accept any baby gifts for the baby before the actual birth of the baby. It's one of those weird religious superstitions that I don't really believe in, like I don't really believe that if you break a mirror you'll have seven years of bad luck. But because this no-planning-for-the-baby weird superstition allows me to be as lazy as I inherently am—"I can't possibly spend time buying anything for the baby. It's my *religion*" and "I certainly can't set up the baby room! I have to go through labor!"—I have become a staunch supporter of the custom.

"I'm thinking of putting duck wallpaper up as a border around the room. What do you think of ducks?" Vivian asked.

"Um, I think ducks are good?" I said.

Vivian, I should also mention, looks fabulous. While my ass gets wider if I even smell food, her butt looks the same as it always has. She still has stick arms and toothpick-thin legs. She was even wearing stiletto heels. The whole Vivian package was making me feel dreadful. How could we bond over pregnancy when Vivian is wearing it so well and seeming to love it? Like models, who can't help but make you feel bad when you're in the same room with them because you know they won the gene lottery, I suppose there are pregnant women out there who just make you feel less than perfect even if they don't mean to. Some women, I guess, won the pregnancy gene lottery.

The dinner was good. I mean, the food was good and the conversation seemed to flow. Although something strange did happen. Shannon and Heather left almost immediately after dinner, professing they were tired, and the others soon followed suit, leaving Vivian and me alone. Granted, my and Vivian's pregnancies did dominate the conversation, and, granted, talk of the pros and cons of daycare and nannies isn't as interesting as talk of new relationships or bad dates, which is what we usually talk about at dinner parties. But I couldn't help but wonder if they thought we were boring. Best not to think that way. Best to think that they really were just tired.

MAY 26

10:00 a.m.

After I got out of the shower this morning and had toweled off, I was walking naked into my bedroom when I caught a glimpse of myself in the full-length mirror. What the heck was that line running down my stomach? Oh my God. That must be a stretch mark. I had no idea what a stretch mark looked like before this morning, but that was the only explanation for the purplish line running from my belly button down to my pubic hair. It was hideous.

I raced back into the washroom to find the vita-min A and E oil that Helena, my aesthetician, had made me buy from her at my last visit. "You have to put this on every day. Just rub a little along your thighs, breasts, and stomach and you won't get stretch marks." I had totally forgotten about doing that. I have, in fact, just got used to taking my Materna vitamin every night.

I poured a handful of the oil into my palm and rubbed it into my stomach, all over the stretch mark. It seemed to work. Phew. Pregnancy Crying Disaster #153 averted. That's the strange thing about pregnancy. You don't really understand what a stretch mark is until you see one, because how are you supposed to know what one looks like?

Varicose veins, however, are a lot easier to see. Helena, as she was giving me a leg wax the last time, was the first to point them out. "You're getting varicose veins. For ten minutes a day, you should lie with your legs higher than your head. That way the blood will flow from your legs and you won't get them." Helena also told me that I must also get a pedicure and bikini wax right before I give birth. "I have a lot of nurses as clients," she said, "and they do make fun of women who have ugly toenails and are bushy Down There. I'm just warning you." I make a mental note to follow all of Helena's advice from now on. I can't have nurses making fun of my chipped pedicure while I'm in labor, that's for sure. That's one more thing I don't want to have to worry about.

The fiancé called and told me we're going on vacation, and not just any vacation. We're going on the best vacation ever, and it's all because of this unborn child.

"I think we should plan a great vacation, maybe in July for two weeks."

"I like vacations," I told the fiancé. "Let me check my calendar. Yep. I'm free in July."

"It's just that everyone has been telling me that we should go away before the child is born, because once the child is born we are never going to have the same kind of vacation again."

"Who are you talking to? Parents?"

"Yes."

"See? This is why I don't like talking to parents. They make everything seem so drastic. So do all these parents you've been talking to always take their children on vacation with them? Or do they just never go on vacation because they have kids?"

"I guess both."

"Um, we don't plan to take our kid on all of our vacations for the rest of our lives, do we?"

"Definitely not."

"Then why would it be our last vacation ever?"

"I'm not sure. But that's what everyone is telling me to do: go on vacation before the baby is born. So let's do it. Let's go on a relaxing vacation. I could use one."

"Okay, no arguments here."

"I'm thinking Hawaii."

"I'm thinking I love you."

"Okay, let me look into it."

Going to Hawaii for Our Last Vacation Ever.
Going to Hawaii for Our Last Vacation Ever,
thanks, apparently, to this unborn child who will
make it difficult for Mom and Dad to go away until
he/she is off to college. I don't really believe this
will be Our Last Vacation Ever, though. Why else
did God invent grandparents and babysitters and
nannies if not to look after your kids when you
go away? Aloha. How do you say "mother" in
Hawaiian?

MAY 28

My mother is turning into Martha Stewart. I went
over to my parents' place for dinner tonight, and
my mother showed me how she's been wasting—I
mean *spending*—her days these last couple of
months. She's been knitting like a madwoman.

"Wow, that's amazing," I told her, as she showed
me this very detailed baby sweater she had finished, with cute little buttons shaped like stars.
"But, okay, don't get mad. Isn't it a little, um,
pink? I mean, what if it's a boy?"

I know people nowadays, it being the twenty-
first century and all, don't like admitting they follow the "pink for girls, blue for boys" rule, but I
couldn't imagine pushing a little boy dressed in a
pink sweater in a stroller. It might be politically

incorrect, but I don't care—I can't put my baby boy in an all-pink sweater.

"Oh, if it's a boy, I'll save it as a gift for someone else."

Phew.

MAY 29

My stomach is so itchy. I can't stand it. Why is it so itchy? Have I got fleas or something? Did something bite me? I don't see any bites. God, can I not have one day where something doesn't go wrong? I'm falling apart here. I really am. Is this what happens when your skin stretches? I . . . can't . . . stop . . . scratching. Need to get my mind off this itchiness. Must think of something else.

MAY 30

Okay, I admit it. I've been thinking of baby names, basically from the moment I found out I was pregnant. One of the more fun things—possibly the only fun thing—about being pregnant is choosing a name for your child. This is a very important decision. Not only will my child be called whatever name I choose for him/her for the rest of his/her life, but I will also have to live with the choice for the rest of *my* life.

I didn't want to bring the whole baby-naming thing up too early with the fiancé. He's still getting used to the idea of having a baby. Plus he's now busy planning Our Last Vacation Ever, and I definitely didn't want to interrupt that. But I did bring it up with him today. It was time. I was going to explode if I couldn't run my names by him. I had a spectacular list of names, and they had to be narrowed down—with his help, of course.

"I've been thinking of baby names. Have you?"

"No."

"Oh. Well, do you want to hear what I have so far?"

"Sure. Go ahead."

"Okay, if it's a boy, I like the name Lyon or Hunter. If it's a girl, I like the names Farrah, Ivy, and Hazel, but I love, love, love the name Apple."

"Apple? Are you fucking crazy?" the fiancé laughed. "Apple? That's a joke, right?"

"No, I love the name Apple. It's original and sounds delicious and it's really pretty and I love apples."

"No way. We are not naming this child Apple. You want our child to go to school and have all the other kids yelling out, 'Hey, Green Apple! Hey, Red Apple!' And what if our child turns out to be a lawyer? Do you think anyone is going to take a lawyer with the name Apple seriously?" A lawyer? When did our four-month-old fetus become a lawyer? Just what the world needs: another lawyer. Sheesh.

"Well, what if our kid turns out to be a writer? It's a memorable name. Apple is a great name for a writer. Or an actress."

"Or a stripper. 'Let's put our hands together for . . . Apple!'" All of a sudden our unborn child went from lawyer to stripper? How did that happen?

"Why don't we just name our son Grapefruit or Mango then?" he continued. "What about Jacob? Jacob is a good, solid name. Jacob is better than Lyon or Hunter."

"Yeah. It's okay. I just know so many Jacobs. It's not very original."

It was clear we were going to need ground rules.

"I veto Jacob," I told the fiancé. "We're allowed to veto each other's choices as often as we want. Are you sure you don't like Apple? Give it a couple of hours. It may grow on you."

"Veto! Veto! Veto!"

"Okay, now you're just making fun of this."

"Hey, it was your rule."

"I'm sorry. Apple is a fantastic name. But let's not talk about this right now. What else is new?"

MAY 31

10:00 a.m.

I decide to keep on the fiancé about names. I had no idea he had such strong opinions on the subject. I thought that since the baby was growing in me he would leave the naming up to me too. It seems fair to me. But it's clear that that is not going to happen. It is also clear that this is going to take a lot longer than I anticipated.

"How about the name Lotus?" I ask.

"No."

"You're not even giving it a chance. You have to say it aloud a few times. Can I at least have a 'Maybe'?"

"Veto."

"Okay, have you given any more thought to Apple?"

"NO!"

"Ryan?"

"I like Ryan."

"For a girl."

"No. Ryan is a boy's name!"

"No, Ryan can be a girl's name."

"Goodbye, Beck."

10:20 a.m.

"Beck? Is that you again?"

"Apple?"

Dial tone.

10:30 a.m.

"What? I'm trying to work here, Beck. Come on!"

"How about Jagger? After Mick Jagger. I love the Rolling Stones, so the name would have meaning. And it could be a girl's or a boy's name. It's perfect. It solves all of our problems."

"I'm on to you. I know what you're trying to do. It's not going to work."

"What? What am I trying to do?"

"You're trying to think of names even more weird than Apple so that Apple will start to sound good to me. It's not going to happen. Apple is not going to happen. And don't you remember what Jason Biggs did to that apple pie in *American Pie*?"

"I am *not* thinking of weird names for weird names' sake." Though that really wasn't such a bad idea. But I have a better idea: I'm going to wait until I'm in the throes of labor, when I'm in so much pain I'm digging my fingernails into his palms, and then scream out, "I want Apple! I want Apple NOW!" He'll have to say, "Yes. Whatever your heart desires." There's no way he'll be able to say no when he sees me in excruciating pain. It would be so rude of him.

"Beck, just do the Stripper Test before you call me up with your next brilliant name suggestion. Just pretend you're the announcer and call out, 'And now, here's . . . Jagger!' See? It's a stripper name."

"I don't like this Stripper Test of yours. Why can't I just pretend I'm calling out the kid's name to get it to come home for dinner or something? The Dinner Test sounds so much better than the Stripper Test and it works just as well."

"Okay. That's fine. Would you feel comfortable calling out, 'Apple! Come home! It's dinner time!'"

"Yes, yes I would. I would be fine with that."

"Enough, Beck. I've got to go. I have a conference call now with some lawyers from Houston."

"Fine. Why don't you ask them if they would do business with a lawyer named Apple? Hello? Hello? Hey, are you there?" Fuck.

1:15 p.m.

"What now? I really don't have time for this."

"Okay, new rule. Let's not discuss baby names until we find out if it's a boy or a girl. That way we'll only have to decide on one name, not two."

"Do you know if it's a boy or girl?"

"No, not yet."

"Are you lying to me?"

"NO!" Of course, that is something I would do. But I wasn't lying. I didn't know.

"I think I can find out next week at the next ultrasound appointment."

"Okay, that's fine by me. Let's not discuss this again until we know if it's a boy or girl."

"One more thing."

"Yes?"

"How about Clover?"

"For what? A dog?"

"No, for our child!"

"I'm hanging up now."

And I thought choosing baby names would at least be fun. I clearly don't have a clue about anything. Maybe I don't know my fiancé as well as I should.

THINGS I DIDN'T KNOW ABOUT THE FIANCÉ
1. He has strong opinions on names.
2. He seems to have quick reflexes—especially when hanging up on me.
3. He has been to a strip joint. How else would he know how the announcers introduce the strippers?
4. He actually works at the office.

THINGS I DO KNOW ABOUT THE FIANCÉ
1. He will always take my call when I call him at work. Even if it means he will hang up on me afterward.
2. I could probably convince him about the name Apple. But I'd have to work very hard at it. Most things I want, the fiancé will give to me, eventually, if possible.
3. He is a very patient man.

JUNE 1

10:45 a.m.

Lena called me early this morning with a Fear Phone Call.

"Oh God. I have The Fear. Last night I slept with a London banker who was in town for business. I think I'm still drunk."

"Do tell. I stayed in watching taped reruns of *Sex and the City*. Tell me everything."

"He was so cute. You'd love him. But he left to

go back to London this morning. He didn't leave me his card or anything, but I gave him my e-mail address. Do you think he'll write?"

"I don't know. Sure, why not?"

"Oh, I hope he writes. He really was sexy. And super nice. I really like him."

We spent the next forty-five minutes discussing the possibility of whether he'd e-mail her or not, and, if he did e-mail her, when that would happen. I tried not to let it bother me that she didn't ask how I was feeling. But it did. Of course, I had nothing to share. Staying home eating potato chips and drinking water is not nearly as interesting as getting drunk and sleeping with a banker from London.

1:00 a.m.

I felt something moving in my stomach. I'm just not sure exactly what it was. But it kept me awake, that I do know. It wasn't exactly a kick, I don't think. It was more like something doing somersaults in my stomach, as though I had eaten a bad dinner or had really bad gas. It was like a fluttering movement. But it wouldn't stop for a long time. Is this what it's supposed to feel like? It was kind of cool for the first five minutes, but I need to sleep!

Cute Single Man surprised me and dropped by my place on his way to work today. He brought me an iced latte. I think he wanted to kiss me. No, I *know* he wanted to kiss me. A girl can tell these sorts of things. I don't know what I'm going to do. I wish I could talk to someone about this. There's no way I can tell the fiancé. I can't tell any of my friends either, because they'll all think it's strange that I have the best fiancé ever (which I do) and I'm hanging out with another man. But Cute Single Man makes me feel good. He makes me feel normal, like life before pregnancy. What is stranger, that I find myself drawn to Cute Single Man and want him in my life or that Cute Single Man is drawn to me and wants to be in my life even though I'm engaged and pregnant with another man's child?

179

The whole day was off-putting, in fact. The arts editor called me this morning and asked me if I could cover a huge outdoor concert which was taking place just outside the city today. I have never turned down an assignment before, but I had to turn down this one. Because of my damn always-full bladder, I have to go to the washroom every five minutes, or at least it *feels* like I have to go to the washroom every five minutes. It's never clear until I actually try to go to the washroom if it's real or a false alarm. When I go out now, I plan my route according to where I know there will be washrooms. I need to know that I will always be able to find a washroom within five minutes of needing one or else it could get very messy indeed. Covering an outdoor concert with hundreds of thousands of people and very few porta-potties would not work for me. How sanitary are porta-potties anyway? Now is not the time to get some weird disease! Plus I haven't had a whole night's sleep for weeks, and I was too tired to figure out how to get there.

I explained the situation.

"Don't worry," said the arts editor. "I'll find someone else to cover it."

This pregnancy *is* changing my life—at least, my bladder is changing my life—and there's not a thing I can do about it.

JUNE 3

It started out as a bad, bad day. I should never have gotten out of bed. I opened my newspaper only to see that my editor had assigned Sexy Young Intern to the concert he had originally asked me to cover. Apparently Sexy Young Intern does not have bladder control issues and is not too exhausted to travel outside the city for the day. She's so perfect she probably never pees. Oh, how easily replaceable I am.

But the day did get better. I still have it. Not only does Cute Single Man want to come over tonight, but this afternoon, as I was walking along the street (yes, to fetch an iced latte), some man checked me out. Rather, he checked out my fabulously natural new big breasts and smiled at me. But then he glanced down and, noticing my bulging stomach, looked away. Still, for a brief second there, I was flattered. Unfortunately, as my stomach gets bigger and bigger, my breasts are starting to look smaller. Well, it was nice while it lasted.

JUNE 4

9:00 a.m.
Today was my second ultrasound appointment—the ultrasound where most women, if they choose to, can find out the sex of their child. I've never contemplated not finding out the sex. I couldn't say no to that piece of information, especially when it was being dangled right there before me. But, unfortunately, my baby was being very stubborn. I just hope that doesn't mean it will take after me in other respects.

"I can't see what the sex is," said the technician. "The baby is holding its legs firmly together right now. Isn't that adorable?"

"No, not really. Give me a second," I said, flicking my stomach with my fingers, much to the horror of the technician.

"What are you doing?" she asked, flinching.

"I'm trying to get the baby to open its legs. I want to know the gender, and I want to know today."

"I'm trying my best. But sometimes they don't want to cooperate. It's just the way it is."

"Well, try harder," I wanted to say to the technician. To the baby I wanted to say, "I'm your mother. Now open your legs!" (a phrase no mother should ever say to her child).

"Well, it doesn't look like we're going to find out anything today. I'm giving up," the technician finally said, taking off her medical gloves.

N-O-O-O!!!

I don't care what the sex is. I just want to know. I had asked Vivian the day before she found out the sex of her child what she was hoping for. "Officially?" she had answered. "I just want the baby to be healthy. I don't care what it is. But, unofficially, I kind of want a girl." The next day, she found out she was having a boy.

Unofficially—and officially—I'm torn. I kind of like the idea of having a boy. Boys seem more independent and don't need to be fussed over as much. Boys like sports, which means that the fiancé would have to spend a lot of time with him doing father-son sporty things, like fishing and football (though I would never tell him this), and Mommy, who doesn't like sports, could nap. Boys also seem easier to keep occupied. Hand them a toy gun or an action figure and you just watch them run around, right? But then I think, Maybe girls are easier. Can't you just hand a little girl a pack of crayons and a coloring book and leave her alone? Aren't girls better in school? Plus baby girls' clothes are so cute. But, then again, so are little baby boys' running shoes. Plus boys always love their mothers, while girls start hating their mothers when they hit the teen years. Yes, I think a boy would be great.

Noon

Actually, a little girl would be great. A mini version of me running around, with long brown hair? Adorable.

12:15 p.m.

I want a boy. Little Puma sneakers and miniature baseball hats? Adorable.

12:17 p.m.

Girl . . .

12:18 p.m.

Boy . . .

Tomorrow I see Dr. G. for my second checkup with him. I'm going to beg him to get me another ultrasound appointment. Though I'm not sure if "I just really want to know the sex of my child" is a good enough reason to get another one so soon. I must think of a list of questions to ask him this time. After five months, I must have *something* I need to ask him about being pregnant.

I've never been so depressed in my entire life. I just got back from Dr. G.'s, and I've gained twenty pounds.

"It's fine. You're doing great," he said.

"But didn't you tell me that you imagined I would gain between twenty-five and thirty pounds throughout my *entire* pregnancy? I'm only halfway finished and I've gained almost that much already!"

"Like I said, we don't worry about small, skinny people gaining weight."

"I guess I should stop eating so many Big Macs."

"Oh, is that your pregnancy food of choice?"

"Yes. A Big Mac a day seems to keep the cravings away."

"Good for you. Enjoy." Gaa! Wasn't he supposed to tell me that Big Macs were bad for me? I couldn't believe this. First he's not overly concerned about my smoking. Now he isn't even going to try to convince me to eat salads instead of crap fast food? Dr. G. is either a pregnant woman's dream come true or a really bad doctor.

I was starting to tear up over my weight gain. I had to get out of there before the tears actually fell.

"Can I get another ultrasound next week? I really want to know the sex of my child, and the baby was being stubborn last time," I managed to get out.

I'm not sure if Dr. G. really didn't mind me

getting another ultrasound so soon or if it was the tears he saw gleaming in my eyes, but he agreed. I can get another one in a couple of weeks.

Of course, I didn't ask him any other questions, as I had planned to do. I just didn't have any questions for him. And I really thought about it, too.

I called the fiancé. I needed him to calm me down.

"I just got weighed at Dr. G.'s. I've gained twenty pounds."

"Really? Wow." Wrong response. Wrong response.

"Don't 'Wow' me. Yes, really! You're going to dump me when you see me." (One of my male friends once told me he thought that, in a relationship, if a woman gained more than fifteen pounds, that would be a deal-breaker for him, and he would break up with her. I wonder if he would include pregnancy weight gain in that.)

I'm not seeing the fiancé for another three weeks, when I plan to go visit him for a week before we head off together to Maui for Our Last Vacation Ever. The fiancé hasn't really seen me with a belly yet. He's going to be shocked. I fear he won't recognize me. I'm going to have to wear a sign around my neck with my name written on it when I get off the plane so he knows who I am, like I'm one of those limo drivers waiting for a client to get off the plane. And I am so sick of people telling me I look "great." It seems to be automatic for everyone to tell pregnant women they look "great," even when I know I do not look "great."

People barely even look at me before saying, "You look great." How is it possible that I look so "great" now, twenty pounds heavier, dressed in sweats all the time, with food spilled all over me? At least the fiancé will tell me the truth. I hope.

"Beck, you're pregnant. You're supposed to gain weight. Did he say everything looked okay?"

"Yes . . . But you don't understand . . ."

"But what? What don't I understand?"

"Something is happening to my ass."

"What do you mean? What's happening to your ass?"

"It's higher, much higher, and way wider. I'm like freaking Jennifer Lopez, except I don't make any money off my butt," I cried. "I have a huge butt now."

"You're being ridiculous. I'm sure you look great." Argh!

"I don't. I really don't."

"I still love you."

"Yeah, yeah. Whatever."

His kind words didn't cheer me up. But a Big Mac probably would. Just like I now know where every public washroom is in this city, I also know where every McDonald's is. I headed over to see my best friend, Ronald, and the light at the end of my depressing tunnel, the Golden Arches.

JUNE 6

Midnight
I'm lying in bed, awake, waiting.

12:03 a.m.
Where's my baby? Why isn't it moving?

12:05 a.m.
Oh, wait . . . yep . . . there it goes. I rub my stomach.

12:47 a.m.
Okay, baby. It's time to sleep now. Sleep! Now! I know you're in there. I wonder if she/he has ears yet.

JUNE 8

I've now officially hit rock bottom. I am a disgusting human being. I am the lowest of the low. I woke up at six in the morning super hungry with no food in my fridge and with the only place open so early—yep—McDonald's. I walked over, in my pajamas, my hair in the messy bun I had gone to sleep with. Walking out of the Golden Arches, armed with an Egg McMuffin and a hash brown, I spotted two colleagues, who are married to each other, running toward me, dressed head to toe in Adidas. What the hell were they doing up so early on Sunday morning? Right—exercising.

I have given up on going to the gym. It puts me in a sour mood. Every time I see a skinny woman running on a treadmill (and they are always skinny), I feel like saying to her, "I hate you." And I do. I hate those women. So this morning I did what any pregnant girl would do upon seeing two non-pregnant colleagues exercising at six o'clock on a Sunday morning: I ran into the alleyway behind McDonald's to hide. I could just picture them going back into the office and telling everyone, "Yeah, we saw Eckler coming out of McDonald's. She looked like shit. Pregnancy definitely does not agree with her." Argh. I am never leaving my apartment again.

3:00 a.m.

LEG CRAMP. LEG CRAMP. What was that? What is happening to me? Why can't I move my left leg? The calf muscle is paralyzed. And excruciatingly painful. My leg is paralyzed! OW! OW! OW! OW! OW! OW! . . . Wait. It's going away. Phew. Must ask Ronnie about that tomorrow. I've never felt anything like that before.

10:00 a.m.

"Oh yeah. Those calf cramps are the worst! The worst," Ronnie said when I called.

"So that's normal?"

"Oh yeah. You have to try to flex through it."

"I can't have that happen again. That was horrifying."

"It just gets worse. Hey, are you feeling the baby move yet?"

"Yeah, every night when I lie down. I actually look forward to it now. And it moves after I eat chocolate: It must be like a sugar rush for the baby. Ronnie? Is it bad that I sometimes purposely eat chocolate just so I can feel the baby moving twenty minutes later? I mean, I know chocolate is bad for my ass."

"Oh God, no. I used to do that all the time. Juice works too. So does coffee. It's the baby equivalent of a caffeine kick."

Sara and I are meeting for hamburgers tonight at a popular diner downtown. She's just entering her french-fry-craving phase. Thank God, she too is craving carbohydrates! She can remain my friend. It's the perfect pregnancy-related friendship, in fact. All my other friends would never think about meeting me for a plate of fries. And I wouldn't dare ask them to, either.

JUNE 10

Sara can't believe I want to find out the sex of my baby. "I'm not finding out. We don't want to know. We figure there are so few surprises left in the world, why not enjoy this one?" she told me when I told her about how my stubborn baby wouldn't open its legs during my last ultrasound appointment.

I can see that, but, really, what's the surprise? It's going to be either a boy or a girl.

Sara also hates the name Apple.

"But," she said, trying to make me feel better, "if I saw Apple Eckler on a menu, I'd order it for dessert. It makes a delicious-sounding dessert." Great.

I don't care. I still love the name.

I'm starting to realize that there are certain things about your pregnancy you should never, ever talk about, not even with your closest friends. Names is one of them. Not because I'm worried that one of my friends is going to steal the baby name (though, I'll admit, that can be a concern. For example, Sara told me last night that she loved the name Ava. I hadn't thought about that name, but I do love it. I love it enough, in fact, to steal it, as I'm giving birth before her), but more because when you share your favorite names with other people, you will never get the exhilarating reaction you're hoping for. And once they turn up their noses at the names you love, they'll want to throw in *their* favorite names, which—trust me—you'll hate.

I was speaking to Heather the other day about possible baby names. I have really started to love the name Ruthie. My grandmother was named

Ruthie. *And* it's a completely *normal* name. I was proud of the name. Until . . .

"Ruthie?" said Heather. "Really? It's so, um, not good for a teenage girl. Isn't it a little, um, grandmotherly?"

"I also really like the name Hazel," I told her.

"Hazel. That's okay, I guess." I can't have an "okay" name for my child. I need the name to be fabulous.

"What about Emily?" suggested Heather.

"Emily? It's okay. It doesn't grab me, though it is pretty."

"You're wrong. Emily is a great name." I never knew there was a right and wrong when it came to baby names, but apparently there is. I'm a failure even when it comes to choosing a good baby name. Apparently.

"How about naming the baby Heather?" said Heather. And this is where it gets really tricky. Even if your friends are joking when suggesting their own names for your child, you never know whether you should take them seriously or not. It happens more than you would ever imagine.

So I've decided not to talk about names before the birth of this child. No matter what, I've realized, someone is going to hate the name I choose. But it's harder for people to scoff at a baby name once there's a real live baby attached to it. That would just be rude. It would be like someone telling me, "I hate the name Rebecca." It just doesn't happen.

11:00 a.m.

Speaking on the phone with Vivian this morning, I casually mentioned to her that none of my friends have been calling to ask how I'm feeling. I told her it was starting to bother me, because I figured she'd understand. Maybe it was happening to her too?

"I noticed that a long time ago. But I don't let it bother me. You have to understand that people's lives don't change just because yours has changed drastically. Everyone always worries about their own problems first. You could call them, you know, and tell them how you're feeling. You shouldn't wait for them to call you. Do you call them to ask how they're feeling?"

"I see your point. But I'm the one who is pregnant."

"You can't let it bother you. Just because they don't ask doesn't mean they don't care. Talk to them about it."

I could never.

Noon

Call from Heather.

"So how *are* you *feeling*?"

"Um, okay. What's new?"

"Oh, nothing. I was just calling to see how *you* are."

1:00 p.m.

Call from Shannon.

"So how *are* you *feeling*? I'm sorry I haven't called recently. I've been super busy at work. So how *are* you?"

1:45 p.m.

Call from Marci, whom I haven't spoken to in a long time. "So how *are* you *feeling*?"

Gaa!!! I'm going to kill Vivian. I really am.

JUNE 16

I knew *Us Weekly* magazine would be more useful than any pregnancy book on the market. I just bought the latest issue and . . . Kate Hudson is pregnant! I'm so excited. It's so much better when you live your life alongside a celebrity's. It makes what you're going through all the more relevant. Plus, Hudson is only twenty-four years old. If a twenty-four-year-old can have a baby and be confident about it, so can thirty-year-old me, right? Right?

Then, coincidentally, just hours later, the fiancé called with a brilliant name for a boy.

"How about Hopper?" he asked. "Sean Penn named his son Hopper, and I really like it."

"Hopper? I love it! I absolutely love it! Wait . . . how did you know Sean and Robin named their child Hopper?"

"Oh, you left one of your old *Us Weeklys* lying around here. I was bored and was flipping through it."

The cover price of the magazine was definitely worth it, much cheaper than the relationship counseling we were headed for over the naming of this child.

"By the way, I found you a baby doctor here. You should call and get an appointment for when you're here in two weeks. I'll e-mail you the number."

"Perfect."

Everything is working out. We have chosen a boy's name, a huge relief. Unfortunately, I just *feel*—and this is just a feeling—that this baby is a girl. Maybe my body is finally talking to me. Joanne, the gym trainer who told me to "listen to your body," would be so proud.

JUNE 17

Under no circumstances can I talk about breast-feeding with another human being. I got in a huge fight with Lena about breastfeeding. I had casually mentioned that I wasn't sure I was going to breast-feed.

"What?! You have to breastfeed. You absolutely must."

I completely understand why women want to breastfeed. But I'm not absolutely convinced it's absolutely necessary. I know that if you breastfeed you basically have to be near your baby every three hours for months on end. Or you can pump, which seems to me excruciatingly painful and so not natural for something that is supposed to be so natural. I just think that if you bottlefeed from the start, then anyone can hold the bottle at any time, day or night. A bottle equals freedom. I had no idea Lena had such strong opinions about breast-feeding. The things you find out about your friends when you're pregnant.

"You have to breastfeed at least for the first lit-tle while. It's so much better for the baby. It really is so much healthier."

"Lena, you've never even been pregnant. How do you know that?"

"I just do. I've read a lot about it and have tons of friends who have had babies." This was begin-ning to sound like a lecture. I was getting annoyed. Who was *she* to lecture *me* about *my* baby and *my* breasts?

"Tons of studies have shown that the nutrients from breastmilk are much better for the baby than formula. Not to mention the bonding that takes place between mother and child during that time."

"Lena! My mother never breastfed and I think my brothers and I turned out fine. In fact, almost none of my friends' mothers breastfed them and they all seemed to turn out okay." I didn't want to tell her that I've seen what has happened to Ronnie's breasts over the past few years, having breastfed three kids. She used to have large, beautiful breasts. Now they're the size of small tomatoes. I didn't want Lena to think I wasn't going to breastfeed because of vanity, however true that may be. It was all I could do to not yell at Lena, "When you get pregnant, you can do what you want. This is my baby, and I'll make my own decision."

"Okay, let's not talk about this," Lena said. I can't believe we fought over breastfeeding, of all things. We almost never fight.

Of course, I have heard that women who breast-feed lose weight a lot faster than women who don't, which is definitely something to think about.

JUNE 20

Total depression. I'm working harder than ever, just to prove I'm still a hard worker, and no one at the paper seems to appreciate my efforts. Sexy Young Intern has also been putting out copy with a vengeance. For every story I write about being in a serious relationship or being pregnant ("Why Renovating Your House Can Lead to Divorce," "Married Couples Who Choose to Live Apart," "Why Even Celebrities Are Eating Fast Food These Days"), Sexy Young Intern writes about, well, being a Sexy Young Intern ("Speed-Dating," "Best Pick-up Lines," "Coolest Bar Patios," "Nifty Summer Beverages"). I feel guilty wanting to be her. Sometimes the feeling is overwhelming.

None of my friends called me tonight to go out because, I'm sure, they're all going to bars, and I don't like going to bars anymore because pregnant women do look strange in bars. It's humiliating. As a pregnant woman you feel you are a downer for all the people trying to enjoy themselves in a bar, trying to pick up the opposite sex. People don't want to sit beside you if they're smokers because they feel guilty about blowing smoke in your pregnant, bloated face. They don't want to get plastered with you because they know you're only drinking water and that makes them feel like lushes. Even my pregnant friends haven't called. They all have husbands they can hang out with. My fiancé called and told me he is going out to a bar with his friends, too. Why wouldn't he? So I called Cute Single Man to ask if he wanted to come over and play Scrabble with me tonight. (Pregnant women can play Scrabble.) He did. He seems to be on call for me. Immediately, I felt better. I'm so grateful that someone still wants to spend time with me, I thought about kissing the guy. I wonder if he is a good kisser.

REASONS TO PURSUE FRIENDSHIP
WITH CUTE SINGLE MAN

1. We have common interests: reality television, movies, Scrabble, Starbucks iced lattes.
2. He calls me, asks how I'm doing, and seems to be interested in hearing the

answer. He seems to want to know everything about my pregnancy.

3. He makes me laugh.
4. It's not every day a Cute Single Man would
   be interested in a pregnant, engaged
   woman.
5. He doesn't seem to care about my "baggage," a.k.a. being pregnant, which makes
   me feel like a normal person.
6. He doesn't seem to care how fat I get.
7. He does stuff for me.
8. Once I move in with the fiancé and have
   the baby, how many other Cute Single
   Man friends will I ever have again?
9. Why not be friends?

REASONS TO NOT PURSUE FRIENDSHIP
WITH CUTE SINGLE MAN

1. It's a little (or a lot) weird that a Cute Single
   Man wants to hang around a pregnant,
   engaged woman. What is wrong with him?
   (Deep, dark, weird obsession or something?)
2. The fiancé would not like it.
3. I would kill the fiancé if he had an equivalent female friend.
4. What if he ends up wanting to pursue
   more than a friendship?
5. What if *I* end up wanting to pursue more
   than a friendship?
6. It is not normal.

I thought I was depressed yesterday. Today the depression continues in full force. I got in a fight with Ronnie today. I never fight with Ronnie. She's too good a person to fight with. She had asked me a simple question about something and I snapped back, "I just don't know. Listen, I can't deal with this right now."

"I can't deal with you," she snapped back. That was when it hit me. I was being a bitch to my best friend, the one friend who has been so helpful every time I've needed her.

"Oh God. I'm so sorry. I'm so sorry. I woke up today and my face is fat!" I started bawling. "I didn't even recognize myself."

While I was washing my face this morning, I noticed it was . . . puffy. My cheeks looked round and swollen, as though I had just had my wisdom teeth removed. I used to have cheekbones. I know I used to have cheekbones. I *remember* having cheekbones. Now my face was like a panda bear's, but definitely not as cute.

"It's okay, Beck. Don't worry. I remember when that happened to me. It's just water retention. It goes down during the day. Are you eating a lot of salty things? Because that sometimes does it."

"I'm so ugly."

"You're not ugly. Trust me. I know exactly how you feel. Once, near the end of my pregnancy, I was meeting a friend I hadn't seen in a while. I got to the

199

restaurant before her and was waiting at the table. I
saw her come in. And you know what she did?"

"No. What?"

"She walked right by me. I had gained so much
weight that she didn't even recognize me! I was so
big, my ankles looked like tree trunks. No joke. I
couldn't even do up my shoelaces. I was wearing
Velcro by the end of my pregnancy."

I started to laugh.

"Really. And I lost all the weight. I lost sixty-
seven pounds. You only have another couple of
months to go."

"No, I have FOUR more months to go. That's a
long time."

"It will go by quickly. I promise."

"Ronnie? I'm so sorry I snapped at you. I'm
just in shock."

"Don't worry. I forgive you. I basically yelled at
everyone when I was pregnant."

"I'm going to find out the sex tomorrow," I told
her, trying to change the subject.

"What's your feeling?"

"I think it's a girl. I just feel it's a girl. But what
do I know?"

JUNE 23

It's a girl! It's a girl! I'm having a girl! I was right.
Maybe my maternal instinct is kicking in. I just
came back from my ultrasound appointment. I

can't believe I was right, though there was a 50-50 chance I would be. The odds were good.

"Do you want to find out the sex?" the technician asked.

That was the only reason I was there, but I didn't want the technician to think I didn't care about whether my baby was healthy or not.

"Sure," I answered, all breezy-like, as if I was leaving a phone message for a guy I had a crush on. Or at least I tried to sound breezy. But I was impatient, and it's hard to sound breezy when you're impatient.

"So, do you know if it's a boy or girl?"

"First I'm checking to see if the spine and heartbeat and all the other measurements are okay. Your baby is very photogenic."

"Really?" Ah, my first feeling of mother-pride! "What do you mean?" Could my baby be pretty enough to be a model? Maybe, one day, this child will not get out of bed for less than $10,000 a day and will be able to support its mother in her retirement.

"Well, I can see everything very clearly. Your baby just yawned."

"It's yawning?" Dear God, is it possible the child is already not a morning person? I wouldn't mind a baby who liked to sleep in.

"Now I'm going to look to see if I can find out the sex for you."

Please, dear baby, open your legs today. Open your legs for Mommy. (That will absolutely be the last time I ever use that phrase.)

"It looks like you're having a girl! I would say 98 percent you are having a girl. I can look up and see the opening between the legs and there is no penis."

I was ecstatic. Unofficially, I really had wanted a girl, aside from the times I had wanted a boy. I grew up with three brothers—one who once tried to shove me in the dryer, another who tried to shove my head in the toilet, and a third who once threw me down on the concrete sidewalk so hard that I had an egg-shaped bump on my forehead for a week. There goes the brilliant name Hopper. But the fiancé and I can now officially start thinking of girls' names. I'm closer to Apple than ever before.

"Hey! It's a girl! It's a girl!" I cried into my phone to the fiancé.

"Really? I knew it. I knew it!"

"Me too! Me too! I knew it too!"

"You did?"

"Yes!"

"Why didn't you say anything?"

"Why didn't you?"

"Because I didn't want you to think I cared whether it was a girl or boy. And I didn't care. Why didn't you say anything?"

"Because I didn't know if you cared one way or the other. So, are you super happy?"

"Yes. Just thinking about a cute little you running around with a ponytail. Plus now I don't

have to get up for early-morning hockey prac-
tices."

"Unless we have a girl who likes to play hockey."

"Then you have to go."

"Do not."

"Do too."

We'll see about that.

The fiancé sent me flowers to congratulate me.
They were very pretty and I officially love him even
more now.

And I now officially waddle, which is not so
pretty.

JUNE 28

10:20 a.m.

Now I officially don't have hipbones either. I know
I used to have hipbones jutting out of my sides. If
I dig my fingers deep into the fat, I can still feel the
bones w-a-a-a-y down there. But I have bigger
worries. Our Last Vacation Ever is fast approach-
ing. In less than a week, I'm going to see the
fiancé, before we head off together for Our Last
Vacation Ever. I haven't seen him since my birthday, six weeks ago. I've warned him to hide any
look of shock, disappointment, or disgust upon
seeing me. But I am even more worried about
bathing-suit shopping, which I have to do for Our
Last Vacation Ever. I can't spend two weeks in
Hawaii without getting into a bathing suit at some

point. I have to go bathing-suit shopping, and I have to get it over with, immediately if not sooner. Maybe it won't be that bad?

12:30 p.m.

Well, that was as expected: awful, awful, awful. On a non-pregnant, skinny day, bathing-suit shopping is painful for almost all women. In fact, I've never had an enjoyable bathing-suit shopping experience. The lighting is always way too bright. (Really, why can't they have the same lighting they have in bars—purposely dark, to hide our flaws?) There are always too many three-way mirrors (because one three-way mirror is one too many three-way mirrors). How can you possibly enjoy looking at yourself in a bathing suit, even the most flattering of bathing suits, when you can see parts of your body you don't, fortunately, see at home? I think shopping for a bathing suit almost six months pregnant is going to lead me to six months of therapy. What I saw was not good, not good at all.

"So can I buy normal bathing suits, just in larger sizes?" I asked the salesclerk immediately upon walking in. I haven't, for a long time, needed to explain that I was pregnant. The bulging belly is there, in full bloom, for the world to see.

"Oh yes. I've had four pregnant women come in already today. They all bought bikinis."

Cool. I am a bikini type of girl.

"And your stomach will look so much better with a tan," she continued. Bonus.

I grabbed a few off the racks—size 12 and they still looked small!—and went into a changing room.

What I saw would scare anyone. Whose ass was that? That most certainly was not my ass. It couldn't be. It looked lumpy and wrinkly, like cottage cheese. GAAA! That must be cellulite. I now have fat *on my back*. How is it possible to get back fat? Who knows? But I have it. Maybe a beach vacation was a mistake. Maybe we should have gone on an arctic cruise or something.

I bought three bikinis, which weren't exactly flattering (I was past the point of hoping for flattering), but at least they covered what needed to be covered. My stomach, hard and round, was now the best-looking part of me.

"Did you find what you needed?" asked one of the employees.

"Sort of. I think I need accessories too."

"What kind of accessories?"

"I need accessories to cover my cottage-cheese butt," I said. "I need a couple of skirts or something."

Six hundred dollars spent on bikinis and accessories to cover up my ass in those bikinis, which I will wear on this vacation only. I must remember to always walk behind the fiancé on Our Last Vacation Ever so he can't see my wrinkly, old man's butt.

4:00 p.m.

A married male writer friend, also the father of an eight-year-old son, called me to check in. He asked what I had been up to, so I told him about my horrific bathing-suit shopping experience.

"Wait. You bought bikinis?" he asked with such scorn you'd think I'd just told him I had been out buying crack cocaine.

"Yes. Why? What's wrong with that?"

"You can't wear bikinis now. You're going to be a *mother*! You have to be modest now."

"What? Because I'm pregnant I can't wear bikinis? That's the most ridiculous thing I've ever heard." Have we not learned anything since Demi Moore posed pregnant and nude on the cover of *Vanity Fair* more than a decade ago? When did all my friends turn so conservative on me?

"What do you want me to wear? A bathrobe to the beach?"

"You should be covering up more."

"I don't tell you how to parent," I told my friend. "So don't tell me what I can or can't wear on the beach."

God, why does everyone have to have an opinion on every pregnant move I make? Even the fiancé is feeling it.

"It's like everyone who has a kid thinks they are experts on parenting," he said. "I went to university, but that doesn't mean I'm an expert on all universities."

"Yeah, well, I can't talk about breastfeeding or baby names to anyone ever again. Because *everyone* has an opinion they can't wait for me to hear."

"Yeah, well, we just have to remember—"

"I know, I know. We just have to remember—"

"How rewarding this will be," we finished in unison.

JUNE 29

7:00 a.m.

As if bathing-suit shopping wasn't enough to drive me to therapy, the fight I got into with the fiancé last night certainly will. I think we have broken up. I have never been so angry with another human being—certainly not with him—ever. How can I possibly forgive him for what he has done to me?

The fiancé has decided to go on a diet. Now, of all times. I called him yesterday, early evening, post cellulite-and-back-fat discovery, when my self-esteem was already at an all-time low.

"I'm buying nuts and seeds," he told me.

"Nuts and seeds? Why? Did you take up birding and forget to tell me?"

"No, they're for me. I went to see a nutrition-ist, after my workout with my new trainer. I'm serious this time about losing weight."

Gaaa!

"You can't be serious," I told him. "Please tell me you're not serious."

"What? Don't you want me to be healthy and fit? I don't want to have a heart attack when I'm forty. I want to be around you for a long time. Don't you want me to be around for a long time?"

"Yes, but I've been supportive of you losing weight for five years and you haven't. Why now, of all times, do you have to go diehard about dieting? I already feel awful enough not being able to control how much weight I'm gaining. And now—*now*—you decide to go on a diet?" That really had come out more bitchy than I'd anticipated.

"Well, what do you want me to do?"

"What do I want you to do? What do I want you to do?" I said, mocking him. "I want you to gain weight with me!" That sounded ridiculous even to my own crazy ears. But it was true. Why does he have to start looking good now, when I'm looking like utter crap? Why couldn't he wait for me to lose weight with him? Why is he trying to impress some nutritionist he just met, when he's never taken my advice about giving up beer and white bread? Is he in love with this nutritionist? I've heard of men who gained sympathy weight when their wives were pregnant. Clearly, my fiancé was not one of those men.

In any case, the fiancé didn't like me mocking him and it went downhill from there. I started screaming that he was in love with his nutritionist and that if he was buying nuts and seeds because of her, he might as well move in with her and marry her and have a baby with her. Then he accused me of being selfish and yelled, "You're always complaining about how fat you're getting, but you're not doing anything about it. You've stopped going to the gym. So stop complaining about how fat you're getting if you're just going to go out and eat McDonald's four times a week," to which I responded that he had no idea how it felt to be pregnant and hungry all the time and not to be able to work out comfortably, and I finished my rant by telling him that he should go to hell. He hung up on me at that point, and I called him back to say, "Don't you hang up on me!" before I hung up on him. Then he called me back and told me I had put him in a miserable mood and he hung up on me for a second time. I'm going to be a single mother. This argument never would have happened if I wasn't pregnant.

10:00 a.m.
Waiting for a groveling call from the fiancé, apologizing to me for deciding to lose weight and get "fit and healthy" now of all times. The nerve.

11:00 a.m.
Still waiting. What kind of man buys nuts and seeds anyway? If I had known he was a nuts and seeds type of guy, I never would have started dating him in the first place.

Noon
I can't believe he's not calling. I'm pregnant! Shouldn't he at least be a little worried about me?

1:00 p.m.
Turning off all my phones so I won't know whether he calls and also so he'll think that I'm

ignoring him, rather than him ignoring me. Two can play at this game. Plus, since he's been eating only "nuts and seeds," he can't possibly be thinking clearly at this point. He has to call eventually.

4:00 p.m.

Ha ha! Just checked my messages. There were three from the fiancé begging me to call, saying that he was getting worried. He's sorry, he said, and he promised not to talk about nuts and seeds ever again. I'm going to wait until seven o'clock to call him. I can't have him thinking I forgive him that easily.

"And you'll be happy to know," he finished his last message, "that I'm going to eat a double cheeseburger for dinner tonight."

Good. He'd better order fries with that.

JUNE 30

Met Vivian today for a coffee. She is one of those pregnant women who really *has* still gained weight only in her stomach. Her arms and legs are still Q-tip skinny. She told me that she and her husband have started taking classes at the hospital to prepare for the birth of their child. They are taking a parenting class *and* a birthing class.

"So what are you learning?" I asked, because, while I am too lazy to actually attend a class, I'm not one for turning down free information. It's kind of like asking a friend for class notes after skipping a class—or a month of classes—in university.

"Last time we learned what the different colors of newborn poop mean," she said.

"Oh. That sounds . . . informative." I was grateful I wasn't the one who had paid to join that class. I mean, really. The baby is going to poop. Is it really that important what color it is?

"We also learned different rocking techniques to use when the baby cries."

"Really? I always thought that when the baby won't shut up, you try everything until it does, including all possible rocking methods."

"Yeah, that's basically what they told us to do."

See? I knew I didn't need to take a class.

JULY 1

I'm now visiting the fiancé at his place. The airport pickup went smoothly—partly because he had been warned dozens upon dozens of times not to look at me with disgust, and partly because before he could even kiss me hello I said, "I know I look bigger, so don't try to convince me otherwise. But this is not permanent. I promise." I suppose that because I had led him to believe that I had gained two hundred pounds, seeing me twenty-something pounds heavier was a relief. "You don't look that bad," he said. "Really, I was expecting so much worse." Still, I made him walk in front of me with my suitcase. I'm not ready for him to see me from behind—even with clothes on—just yet.

"Do you think I can get away with wearing your baggy T-shirts and a pair of sweats the entire vacation?" I asked him.

"Sure. Why not."

"Okay, good. Because that's what I'm planning on wearing, since barely anything from last summer fits."

I now understand why some people suggest you hide away all your pre-pregnancy clothes as soon as you know you are pregnant. Some things are best forgotten about. Like losing your virginity. It's better to repress memories that aren't as fond as they are supposed to be.

JULY 3

The fiancé was at work all day today, so I spent my day doing what I always do when he's working and I'm staying with him: I called Lena for a long chat. I've given up on her asking how I'm feeling, because I realize it's just not her style. The less you expect of other people, the easier it is. Instead, I've decided to take a new approach. I'm just going to jump in and talk about myself once in a while.

"Lena. You don't understand. Last night we were watching television and I went to crawl up on his lap, like I always do when we watch TV together. And you know what he said?"

"What?"

"He said, 'OW!' He actually said, 'OW!' I really hurt him when I climbed on him! That's how heavy I'm getting."

"I don't believe it."

"Believe it. I can't get used to this body. I won't even let him see or feel me naked. I fear he won't be attracted to me and won't be able to get it up, and that will make me feel even worse! Can I go until October not having sex with my fiancé? Maybe I can tell him the doctor told me 'no sex.'"

"Don't forget you can't have sex for at least a month after giving birth."

"Thanks for reminding me, Lena. What am I going to do?"

"Some men find pregnant women very sexy. There's a ton of porn websites about pregnant women. Maybe he finds you sexier than ever?"

"Okay, I'm not sure how you even know about those websites and I'm not going to ask. But I don't think he finds me super sexy. He doesn't make any passes at me in the bedroom, either."

"Don't worry about it. He loves *you*. Which means he loves you just as you are. He knows you're pregnant and that your body had to change. If anything, he probably thought you were too skinny before. And he's a *guy*! He will want sex no matter what."

Maybe Lena is right. Maybe I could still have sex with my fiancé.

"You *are* going to lose all the weight," she continued. "And if it's harder than you think, you'll just have to take drastic measures."

"What? You mean liposuction?"

"No, you'll have to get him to send you to a fat farm for a couple weeks."

Oh. Right.

JULY 4

The fiancé and I stopped at the drugstore today to get some supplies. Driving home, the fiancé caught me tearing up.

"What now? What's wrong?"

"The song."

"The song on the radio? What about it?"

"It's just . . . it's just so sad."

"Phil Collins? I didn't even know you liked Phil Collins."

"Me neither. But it's so sad."

"You're not going to be like this on our vacation, are you?"

"I don't think so. I hope not." At least I wasn't crying over long-distance TV commercials.

"Good. Because it's—"

"I know," I said, cutting him off, "Our Last Vacation Ever."

Later, we both made a horrible mistake. We

were bumming at his place, flipping channels, just as a birth show was about to start on one of those women's networks.

"Hey, have you seen one of these shows before?" I asked him.

"No. Have you?"

"No. Maybe we should watch it. They're supposed to make you feel all warm and fuzzy about having a baby. Maybe it will be good for us? Maybe it will make us feel all warm and fuzzy. Maybe we'll finally understand how 'rewarding' this will be."

Maybe not. Definitely not. We lasted exactly four and a half minutes before we had to turn off the TV. We didn't even witness a woman giving birth. All we saw was the obstetrician stick his hand up a woman to see if she was dilating. We didn't see anything but the outside of this woman's thighs. She wasn't even naked. She was wearing a hospital gown that covered all her private parts.

"I can't watch this," I told the fiancé, which was weird. I have had many Pap smears done. Getting a Pap smear is no trip to Disneyland, but it's not usually mortifying. But watching someone else have a doctor stick his hand up her—even if we couldn't really see anything—made both of us super queasy.

"I can't watch this either. Please, let's turn it off," the fiancé begged.

I looked over at him. He looked pale. I'm not sure how any woman can be addicted to shows like these, though I know there are lots who are. I don't think the fiancé will be able to last during delivery. I don't think *I* will be able to last during delivery, and that's a really big problem.

JULY 6

In bed last night, I asked the fiancé about something that's been bothering me ever since I arrived.

"Is your bed smaller, or is it just me?" The fiancé has always had the most comfortable, huge, king-size bed. I used to look forward to crashing in it. But suddenly I was claustrophobic lying there. He seemed so close. And I seemed to be tossing and turning more.

"Maybe you're just bigger so it seems smaller," he suggested.

"Thanks. Thanks a lot."

"You know what I mean."

JULY 7

The fiancé drove me this morning to see an obstetrician in his city. We haven't fully decided where I will give birth yet, but I have decided that I can't give birth vaginally. I have been having panic attacks about once a week where I wake up with a start and have a hard time breathing when I think about going through labor. The thought of a baby coming out from Down There terrifies me. How can a baby possibly come out from Down There? This is not the eighteenth century. I'm not a farm woman who has to give birth on a wooden table. I'm a modern career woman who barely has time to schedule a manicure.

I had already asked Dr. G. if he does scheduled C-sections. I once read an article about celebrities and powerful New York career women who are "too posh to push" and who book C-sections like they book dentist appointments. It sounded ideal to me. You know exactly when you are going to give birth—"Next Tuesday? Sorry. I can't meet you for lunch. I'm having a baby. What about Wednesday?"—and there would be no fear of having your water break in public, no possibility of a long, painful labor, no post-birth hemorrhoids, and no worry about the fiancé seeing me in the most humiliating position ever (legs spread wide, sweat pouring off my face, me swearing like a sailor). I've also heard that C-section babies come out looking prettier, without the dented heads common to babies who come out from Down There. I want my baby to come out pretty.

"No, you can't schedule a C-section. We don't do that," Dr. G. told me. "Maybe in Brazil they do that, but not here." Damn.

I had lies prepared for this obstetrician, Dr. Bono. I call him that because his accent reminds me of Bono from U2.

Dr. Bono is very different from Dr. G. He's about fifteen years younger, and he wasn't dressed in scrubs, like Dr. G. always is. He was dressed in black slacks and a slick dress shirt, and he had a full head of curly hair with product in it. He looked like a wannabe movie star. I am weirdly attracted to him. He's a hot doc. Of course, it could be my pregnant hormones.

"I was wondering if Dr. B. does planned C-sections?" I asked the nurse. "I'm having awful panic attacks about giving birth. I don't think I can do it. I really am that scared. I wake up crying every night because I'm so worried about giving birth." I had to test drive my lies/lines on someone.

"I'm not sure. You'll have to ask him. But maybe you should think about taking a birthing class so you'll know what to expect," the nurse suggested. "That might make the experience easier."

"I suppose I could do that," I told her, though I knew that was never going to happen. I know enough to know I'd rather not know anything.

"Dr. B. will be right in," she said, leaving the room.

Be a good actress, I told myself. You can be a good actress.

Dr. B. entered the room and I launched into my prepared speech with a flourish.

"Listen. I'm going to tell you right off the bat that I can't give birth. There's no way. I wake up every night with panic attacks. I can barely breathe and I can't sleep anymore because I am so worried about giving birth. I know I can't do it, and I will do anything if you could please schedule me a

C-section. I will even think about naming my child after you—that's how serious I am about not being able to give birth vaginally," I spewed out, blinking my eyes rapidly as if I was trying to hold back tears. And the Oscar goes to . . .

"Sure, I can do that. No problem," said Dr. B. in his Bono-esque accent.

What? Excuse me?

"Really?"

"Yeah. It's not a problem. We'll schedule one the next time you come in for an appointment. To tell you the truth, I'm not sure why more women don't request them. The whole operation should take about twenty minutes. I still have to give you an epidural, though. You won't feel anything from just below your breasts to your thighs."

Twenty minutes? I could fit that into my schedule. It sounded fantastic and too good to be true.

"Can I just be asleep for the whole thing?"

"Ah, no. I won't do that." Well, I had to ask.

"Well, will there be a curtain up so I don't have to see what you're doing to me?"

"Of course. We're not going to make you watch," he laughed.

And that's when I fell in love with Dr. Bono and decided that I will have my baby in the fiancé's city with Dr. Bono, who will give me a C-section.

Excited that I found a doctor who would do a planned C-section for me, I couldn't wait to share the good news with all my friends. Not even the fact that Dr. Bono told me I'm now twenty-five pounds heavier than my pre-pregnancy weight could dampen my spirit. I called Ronnie first.

"Guess what?" I told her. "I found a doctor who will do a planned C-section. Isn't that great?"

"What? Are you crazy? You can't do it. The recovery time is so much longer. It's major surgery. You should never do a C-section unless you have to. It can be dangerous."

"But a lot of women do it," I told her. "What about all those women who go through twenty hours of labor only to get a C-section at the end? What about all the celebrities who get C-sections?"

"They cut through all your stomach muscles. You won't be able to hold your baby after because you'll be in too much pain. You will barely be able to breathe. And you won't be able to work out for weeks after because it will hurt even to walk. And forget about breastfeeding. It will be too painful."

I could see it was definitely not the right time to tell Ronnie that I wasn't positive I was going to breastfeed either. I feared she would go into convulsions. But Ronnie did give me something to think about. I do want to start working out immediately after giving birth. I'm going to have to give this C-section more thought.

2:00 p.m.

I can see how Ronnie might not agree with planned C-sections, Ronnie being one of those mothers who believes she is a hero for giving birth vaginally. I do not need to give birth vaginally as a badge of honor. But I was shocked at my friend Shannon's reaction. Shannon is a modern woman whose career comes before all else. She reads all the latest magazines and keeps up with current events. She wears only black.

"Well, that's not very feministic of you," she said when I told her I could have a planned C-section if I wanted.

"Feministic of me? What do you mean? I have to go through vagina pain to be a feminist now? Is that in some Gloria Steinem book I missed?"

"Yes. Women have been having babies for centuries and centuries. Why are you being so spoiled about it? Giving birth is a beautiful experience and you're turning it into a chore you can get out of. This is the one thing that men can't do. Giving birth is what makes us stronger than men. It's the ultimate self-sacrifice."

"Oh. I hadn't thought about it that way," I told her. Her vehemence was scaring me. "Well, I haven't made a decision about it yet. I just like having the option."

Am I a bad feminist? And do I really care? I mean, isn't feminism all about having choices, the freedom to make your own decisions?

4:00 p.m.

I can't get the whole C-section-versus-vaginal-birth thing off my mind. I think I might actually have to find out exactly what happens during labor before I make my decision. I need to know *exactly* what it feels like and what the aftermath of birth is really like. I need to know the truth. I call Ronnie back.

"You have to wear diapers after," she says.

"What?"

"You have to wear huge maxi pads for a couple of weeks after because gunk keeps pouring out of you."

Score 1 for a C-section.

"No no no no no. That can't be possible. I'm not a maxi-pad kind of girl. I'm a tampon kind of girl. Are there special diapers or something for post-birth?"

"No. You don't literally have to wear diapers. But you can't wear tampons for a couple months after."

Score 2 for a C-section.

"What else?"

"Hemorrhoids. They're like little balloons coming out of your bum."

"No no no no no. That can't be possible."

"Oh, it's true. And they are very painful. I didn't even know what they were until I was in the shower and felt these awful things coming out of me. I thought they had screwed something up during labor. It was so embarrassing."

Definitely leaning toward a C-section. Definitely.

"Okay, but tell me what labor is like. What's it

like when the baby is coming out? Is it super painful? Tell me the truth. I need to know."

"No, really, it's not that bad. I was basically laughing the first time I was in labor. Just make sure you get the epidural and it will be fine."

How could she have been laughing through labor? Every time I've seen a woman give birth in a movie or on TV she's moaning and crying and screaming and swearing. Ronnie must have repressed the whole experience.

"The worst is getting the epidural. That's the most painful part. They sometimes have a hard time finding the right place on your spine to put the needle in."

"Do not say the word 'spine' to me. I hate that word. Ewww. It makes me tense just hearing it."

"You have to lie totally still on your side when they do it, so every time you have a contraction, they have to stop and wait until you're still again to try and get the needle in your . . . you know what. But the worst is that you can kind of hear this weird crunching sound as the needle goes in."

"Okay. Stop! STOP! You have to stop. I can't take this anymore."

"It's really not that bad," Ronnie continues. "That's the worst part. The labor is nothing. Really."

Hmmm. Maybe I could do it vaginally if the worst part is getting the epidural.

"You could also get a doula. I had one for child number three and it was an amazing experience."

"What exactly does a doula do?"

"Well, she becomes your best friend before and during birth and will answer all your questions. She will massage your vagina to loosen it up so the muscles will be relaxed before you pop."

"What? Did you just say she'll massage my vagina?"

"Yep. It really helps."

"No no no no no. I can't have anyone massaging my vagina. That's nasty. And I probably won't have any questions."

"Trust me. By the time you are in labor, so many people have seen your vagina that it's not even yours anymore. You won't care."

Oh yes I will. No one is massaging my vagina.

5:00 p.m.

"I forgot to mention one more thing about the birthing process," Ronnie says, calling me back.

"It better not be bad. I don't want to hear it if it's bad."

"Okay, I'm not going to tell you then. Forget I called."

"No, tell me."

"Well, some women, um, poo during labor."

"No no no no no. That can't be true."

"Yes, it is. You can't control the muscles Down There."

"I don't even know how to respond to that. So I'm going to go now and pretend this little conversation never happened."

"Well, you're the one who wanted to know everything. I'm just trying to help."

Can giving birth be any more disgusting?

JULY 11

We've made it to Maui for Our Last Vacation Ever. So far, Our Last Vacation Ever is heavenly.

JULY 12

I'm even walking around in my bikini. No one but the fiancé knows me here, so I don't care. But I am still making sure I walk a little behind him so he can't see my butt.

JULY 13

Heaven . . . The fiancé is letting me eat whatever I want. It is, after all, Our Last Vacation Ever. I've booked myself a pregnancy massage at the hotel spa. I told the fiancé my back was starting to hurt—and it is. Maybe the massage will help.

4:00 a.m.

"Baby?" I say to the fiancé. "I can't sleep."

Hmmm. He's not hearing me.

"Hey! Why did you just poke me? That hurt."
Now he's awake.

"I can't sleep."

"Why? Is something wrong?"

"My stomach hurts. I think I can feel it
stretching."

"Should we go to the hospital?"

"No," I say, starting to laugh. "I think my stomach is just growing. I can feel it growing. Hey . . .
are you awake?"

"Sorry. I fell back to sleep. Is there anything I
can do?"

"No. Just go back to sleep. Don't worry about
little old me." I'm thirty years old and I'm having
growing pains.

6:00 a.m.

Haven't fallen back to sleep. My stomach hurts.
Poor me. I really can feel my sides stretching out.
The body is not meant to have something growing in it. It's just not. And how exactly did the
fiancé fall back to sleep so quickly? This is the
most time we've spent together since finding out
I was pregnant.

He did seem to get a kick out of feeling the baby
move the first time. But the novelty of that seemed

to wear off quickly. He's not as patient as I am. Whenever I tell him the baby is moving and he goes to put his hand on my stomach, the baby stops moving.

"Did you feel that? Did you feel it?" I ask him as I race to grab his hand and place it on my stomach.

"I think so."

"Keep your hand there. Come on, baby. Move for your papa," I'll say to my stomach.

"Whoa! I felt that. Was that the baby?"

"Yeah, isn't it cool?"

"Yeah. That's cool," he'll say, kind of dreamily. Or maybe he says it in awe, as if he still can't believe that I'm really pregnant and that there's a little human growing in me. And then he'll go back to watching television.

At least we are enjoying the relaxing aspect of this vacation. All we do is watch television, lie by the pool or on the beach, and read magazines. And the fiancé doesn't ever seem to get sick and tired of going through the C-section-versus-vaginal-delivery debate with me. We even had sex yesterday afternoon. I made him turn all the lights off and shut the blinds so it was pitch black. But still. I've missed being intimate. And—phew—he obviously still finds me somewhat attractive. And although I can't move around as easily as I used to be able to, the sex was a success.

9:00 p.m.

The fiancé and I just got back to the hotel room after a relaxing dinner when I felt something I have never experienced before.

"I have this weird burning in my throat. And my heart feels like it's burning. But it's mostly burning in my throat," I told the fiancé. "It hurts to swallow. It's like someone lit a match against my throat."

"Heartburn," said the fiancé.

"Heartburn? Is that what heartburn feels like?"

"Yep. Let me get you a tablet. Welcome to my world."

I always thought heartburn was a middle-age thing. Nothing sexy about heartburn.

A trip to the ice cream store turned into a huge disaster. How is something as easy as a trip to the ice cream store a possible disaster? When you're pregnant, anything is possible.

The fiancé and I had a lovely, romantic dinner in a restaurant in a mall in Maui. "You know, I kind of feel like an ice cream cone. I saw an ice cream shop downstairs," I told him. He was in a good mood too. Even though I had already had an ice cream cone at lunch, he agreed to buy me another. As we walked into the shop, the woman behind the counter pointed to my belly and said, "Hey, I see we have two girls coming in."

"Wow. How did you know I am having a girl?" I asked, amazed.

"Women who are going to have girls carry all the weight in their behinds," she answered.

Oh. My. God. Bitch.

"So what can I get for you?"

"Um, well, now that I know for a fact my ass is big, nothing, thank you," I said.

"Don't worry, I'm sure your man loves a gal with a big behind."

Gaaa! This woman should be fired.

"So what will it be?"

"Um, really, nothing. Goodbye."

The fiancé can now tell when I'm about to cry, and I was about to cry.

"Beck, don't listen to her. She's just a silly woman who works in an ice cream shop in a mall. You can't take what she says seriously."

I couldn't help it. I started to sob.

I told the fiancé I'm never eating ice cream again.

THINGS PEOPLE SHOULD NEVER SAY TO PREGNANT WOMEN—EVER

1. "You look healthier," which is just another way of saying they can tell you've gained weight.
2. "Are you carrying twins?" which is just another way of saying, "You look like you're carrying twins."
3. "No, your ass is not bigger," which is just another way of saying, "I'm lying to you."

4. "It's nice to see your plate full," which is just another way of saying, "Wow. You're eating a lot."
5. "Your face looks different," which is just another way of saying, "Hey, didn't you used to have bone structure?"

JULY 16

Eating Oreo cookie ice cream and loving it. My ass is already fat, so who cares? Plus, the sun is shining and I'm lying on a beach. I'm happy. Why shouldn't I live it up? We're on vacation. No one can see my ass when I'm lying down anyway.

JULY 17

Rough, rough night last night. At two o'clock, I woke up with the worst stomach cramp I have ever experienced in my life. It was so bad, I felt like I was about to throw up. I grabbed the fiancé's hand hard, waking him up. "OW. Cramp. OW OW OW OW! Something's happening." I could barely breathe.

"What's wrong? Should we go to the hospital?"

"Wait . . . wait . . . Oh my God." And then it passed. The whole thing lasted thirty seconds.

"Are you okay?"

"I think it might have been one of those false contractions. I think they're called Braxton Hicks. I saw that happen to Rachel on *Friends.*"

"Are you okay now?"

"Yes. But if that's what real contractions feel like, there's no way I can go through labor. No way. I'm getting a C-section for sure."

"I think that's a good idea."

I stayed up for hours after, fearful that it would happen again. It didn't. Thank God. I mean, I didn't want to ruin Our Last Vacation Ever by going into early labor.

JULY 18

The fiancé and I made another awful mistake. It rained today and we had to kill time, so we went to the hotel's business center to play around on their computers. Damn modern technology is all I have to say. We typed "C-section" into a search engine and checked out pictures of the operation. There should be warnings attached to sites that graphically show photos with step-by-step descriptions of how an operation is performed. There's a reason I'm a writer and not a doctor.

Ronnie is right. Basically they do remove your stomach and plop it on the table beside you before they take the baby out. And then they put your stomach muscles back in and stitch you up.

It really did look painful. But we couldn't turn away. It was like watching a train wreck.

"Did you see all that blood?" I moaned to the fiancé, who finally shut down the computer. "I can't do that. There's no way I can go through that. I didn't know it was possible for there to be so much blood from one operation."

"Well, have you ever seen pictures of vaginal birth?" the fiancé asked.

"No. And I don't plan to after seeing that."

"Unfortunately, I think it will be just as painful but in a different way."

He has a point. I can't do it. I can't have this baby come out of me either by C-section or out from Down There. That's it. This baby isn't coming out of me ever. Period.

JULY 24

A tank top that I wore I'm sure only yesterday no longer fits over my belly. How long exactly have I been asleep?

BAD THINGS ABOUT BEING PREGNANT
1. Uncontrollable gas. I have to live with the embarrassment of farting in front of the fiancé. He thought it was funny. I did not.
2. Uncontrollable eating binges.
3. Uncontrollable emotions.

4. Uncontrollable weight gain.
5. Varicose veins.
6. Wrinkly ass which you have to hide from your fiancé.
7. Back fat.
8. No drinking/smoking/sashimi.
9. Itchy stomach skin.
10. Hyperactive bladder.
11. Leg cramps.
12. Not fitting into any old clothes.

NICE THINGS ABOUT BEING PREGNANT
1. Floating in the swimming pool more easily.
2. People hold doors open for you. Sometimes.

JULY 25

Our Last Vacation Ever is now o-v-e-r. The fiancé is back at his home, and I'm back at mine. I miss him horribly. By the end of our vacation, I even let him walk behind me. I'm planning to marry the guy one day, and we're going to have to abide by the "for better or worse" part. My ass is the "worse" part now. Plus, I think he enjoyed being around me while I was eating like a pig. It allowed him, too, to eat like a pig, without the guilt.

I had another doctor's appointment with Dr. G. today.

"Wow, look at how big you've gotten," he said when I walked into the examining room.

Um, was an obstetrician supposed to say that to one of his pregnant patients? I was pretty certain it wasn't a good thing that an obstetrician—a man who sees only pregnant women day in and day out—seemed shocked at how large I was. Was it possible I looked abnormally large compared to other pregnant women?

"What? Is it bad? Am I gaining too much weight?"

"So far you've gained thirty pounds. That's definitely on the higher side, but I'm not worried. It's just that I always thought of you as a tiny person and now you're not."

Enough!

"The only downside to your gaining this much weight is that there is a greater chance you will get stretch marks," he continued.

Could this appointment get any worse? I still have three months to go.

I called the fiancé to tell him what the doctor had said to me.

"Well, he said everything looked okay, right?"

"Yes. But I still have three more months to go and I've already gained more weight than some women gain during their entire pregnancies."

"Wait. There are only three more months left?"

"Yes. I'm going into my third trimester."

"God, we really have to get our shit together. We have so much to do. We still have to get a night nurse and a nanny, baby furniture and a stroller and a car seat, and all the other supplies we don't even know about."

"I know," I said, cutting him off. He was starting to stress me out. "People told me that I would enjoy the second trimester more than the first. I haven't. People told me that I would get my energy back this trimester. I haven't. People told me that I would get horny this trimester and that hasn't happened either, as you are well aware. Who are these women who get horny and enjoy the second trimester?"

"Well, we did have an amazing vacation. So let's try to enjoy the final three months. After all, these are our last months of freedom."

Thanks for reminding me. In three months I will have a baby and will be living in a new city with the fiancé for the first time ever. And we still need a freaking baby name. And I have to decide whether I want a C-section or not, whether I want to breastfeed or not, how much maternity leave I want to take, if I want to take any at all. I have to end my "relationship" with Cute Single Man. I have to make sure Sexy Young Intern doesn't get my job. It's as though I've accomplished nothing in the past three months. It's as though the only things that have made any progress are my stomach and butt, my "relationship" with Cute Single Man, and Sexy Young Intern's career.

"Do you remember anything about these last three months?" I asked the fiancé. "They seem like such a blur to me."

"All I remember is you asking, 'Is my ass fat?' 'Is my ass fat?' 'Is my ass fat?'"

I didn't want to break it to the fiancé that I had heard the second trimester was the most uneventful of all the trimesters. If these past three months were supposed to be the "easy" months, we're in big, big trouble.

THE THIRD (AND FINAL!) TRIMESTER

a.k.a. The Even Fatter Months

JULY 27

6:15 a.m.

The itsy-bitsy spider went up the . . . went up the . . . went up the something-something. I'm not sure how or why it happened this morning, but I awoke with a jolt, breathless, with this stupid nursery rhyme on my brain. Or, rather, I woke up desperate to remember the words to this stupid nursery rhyme. I can't recall what the itsy-bitsy spider did, and it's driving me nuts. I can't fall back to sleep now. Not before I figure out what the damn spider did. It's like having a well-known actor's face pop into your head and not being able to remember his name, or like trying to remember the name of your Grade 3 teacher when you're twenty-seven, or like trying to figure out what happened to that great sweater that you haven't seen for months and that isn't in your closet. It's driving me crazy. *The itsy-bitsy spider went up the . . . went up the . . . went up the something-something.* What the heck did the itsy-bitsy spider go up? Or did the itsy-bitsy spider go down? Gaa! Will I need to know, in three months, what happened to the itsy-bitsy spider? How can I possibly be a good mother if I can't remember the itsy-bitsy spider song? How is my baby supposed to thrive when she has a mother who can't remember the words to "The Itsy-Bitsy Spider"? Never mind the fact that I have an awful, awful voice.

6:18 a.m.

This little piggy went to the market. This little piggy went to . . . Where did the second little piggy go? Did he go to the zoo? Did he go to the superstore? Did he go to the spa? And where did the third and fourth little piggies go? I know the last little piggy went " 'Waa waa waa' all the way home." But what the heck did the other pigs do? I'm not going to freak. Maybe my kid won't need to know what happened to the other piggies. How important can it be to know where the second, third, and fourth piggies went? It's not exactly information that can get my kid into Harvard, is it? But how can I have forgotten what happened to the piggies? I'm going to be a bad, bad mother.

6:19 a.m.

Twinkle, twinkle little star, how I wonder where you are . . . dah, dah, dah, dah, dah, dah, dah, dah, dah, dah, dah, dah, dah . . . Twinkle, twinkle little star, how I wonder where you are. I'm going to totally *suck* at this mother thing—I can't even remember the words to "Twinkle, Twinkle Little Star"! I do, however, know all the words to Madonna's early songs—"Get into the Groove" and "Like a Virgin," for example—and I can also hum theme songs to many old television shows, like *Beverly Hills 90210,* but that does not a good mother make. Argh.

6:21 a.m.

Who would know the words to these nursery rhymes? Is it too early to call Ronnie?

6:22 a.m.

"Hi. It's me. I know you're still sleeping, but can you call me immediately? Something bad has happened. I need to talk to you ASAP."

6:24 a.m.

"Did you just call me?" the fiancé asks groggily. "I thought I heard my phone ring."

"Yes. I just left you a message. Didn't you get it?"

"No. But who else would be calling me at this hour? What's wrong?"

"I can't remember what happened to the second and third little pigs, and I can't remember the middle verses to 'Twinkle, Twinkle Little Star.'

Do you know if the itsy-bitsy spider went up or down, and if so, what the hell did it go up or down?"

"Beck, what the heck are you going on about now?"

"Nursery rhymes! I can't remember any of them. Can you?"

"Beck! It's 6:30 in the morning your time. Couldn't this have waited until I at least had a coffee or a shower? Or forever?" I had forgotten about the time difference. It's 4:30 in the morning for the fiancé.

"I'm going to be an awful mother. Awful."

"No you're not. I'm sure we can buy a CD with nursery rhymes on it. I can't believe you're worried about this. Furthermore, I can't believe you're worried about this at this hour. Furthermore, I can't believe you're even awake to worry about anything at all at this hour."

"I hadn't thought about getting nursery rhymes on a CD. But that's true. I'm sure someone has put nursery rhymes on a CD. Or maybe we can download them from the Internet. Maybe I won't be an awful mother after all."

"If there's one thing I'm not worried about it's you being a good mother. I'm positive you're going to be a great mother."

"Really?" The fiancé has never shared that with me before. How can he have such confidence in my so-far nonexistent mothering skills? I kill plants! I don't own a frying pan! Change diapers?

Feed a baby? Soothe a baby? I don't know how to do any of it.

"Really. You're going to be great. I know you're going to be great. Now can I please go back to bed? *Please?*"

"Yes. Yes. I'm sorry. I'm just freaking a little."

"I'll call you later, okay? Love you."

6:45 a.m.

"What *now?*" the fiancé answers, this time not so much groggily as angrily.

"I just remembered something. *Mary had a little lamb, little lamb, little lamb. Mary had a little lamb whose fleece was white as snow,*" I sing to him. "Aren't you proud of me?"

"I'm going back to bed," the fiancé says, hanging up on me.

Phew. Now I can sleep too. I may not know what the itsy-bitsy spider did, but at least I know that Mary had a little lamb whose fleece was white as snow. My memory hasn't completely let me down.

JULY 28

Noon

I have just come back from the corner store. I have bought a pack of cigarettes, which I will not, under any circumstances, open. I had planned on buying a carton of ice cream. But on the way to the store, while I was waiting at a red light to cross the street, a woman standing beside me on the corner asked how far along I was.

"Six months," I answered. She was looking at me with such an eerie, uncomfortable expression on her face that I had to ask, "Are you okay?"

"Yes, sorry. It's just that I had such a painful delivery that whenever I see a pregnant woman I get the urge to cross my legs," she responded.

"Really? How old is your baby?"

"Oh, he's not a baby anymore. He's twelve! I'm sure you'll have no problem, but I was in labor for twenty-four hours," she added, shivering at the memory.

I must have had a horrified look on my face. Twelve years since she gave birth and she still gets the urge to cross her legs upon seeing a pregnant woman? Twenty-four-hour labor? It must have been really awful. Her urge to cross her legs upon seeing pregnant me made pregnant me want to smoke with a vengeance.

I will not open the pack of cigarettes. Well, maybe I'll take two drags from one cigarette. And then I'll throw the pack down the toilet for sure.

12:20 p.m.

Heaven. I took four drags and threw the rest of the cigarette in the toilet. Is it possible my baby can crave a smoke? I hid the rest of the pack under the cushion in my couch, just in case I run into that woman again. I have no willpower. Obviously. So, hopefully, out of sight, out of mind.

The fiancé and I have still not decided—rather, I have still not decided—whether to go the C-section or the vaginal route. We still have time. Like any decision, whether it be where to go for vacation or what movie to rent, the more time you have to think about something, the more difficult the decision gets. Especially when information keeps being thrown at you.

One of the fiancé's friends told him that she had a masseuse come into the delivery room with her. Apparently, you can pay anyone to do anything for you these days. This masseuse massaged her back all through labor, and, supposedly, this woman had a great labor that lasted only four hours, which still seems like an excruciatingly long time to me but which in labor-land is supposedly an extremely short period of time. Still, getting a four-hour massage does sound amazing.

Ronnie told me that many of the mothers in her book club had doulas with them during their labor. A doula is kind of like a personal assistant, except instead of answering your phone and replying to your mail at the office, a doula will talk to the doctor for you, fetch you ice chips, and basically make the experience as pleasurable—and as easy—as possible. *If* it's possible that labor can be pleasurable or easy. I'm still not convinced.

"If we go the vaginal route, we should think about hiring a doula," I tell the fiancé.

"Okay, I've heard of Doula. I'll set that up for you if you want. Maybe I'll call and find out more. Do you have a number?"

"I'll ask around. It will take the pressure off you, too. Because the doula can rub my back and yell at the doctor to get me drugs when I'm in pain. She'll know exactly what to do. You kind of hurt me when you give me a massage anyway."

"I do not hurt you. I give great massages. But, okay, get her number."

"First I have to find one."

"Find who?" the fiancé asks.

"The doula."

"Don't you know her number? Can't you get it from Ronnie?"

"Ronnie will be able to find me a doula's number, I'm sure," I tell the fiancé.

"What? If you already know about Doula, then it should be easy to get her number."

"What?"

"Beck, why do you keep 'what'-ing me? Get me Doula's number and I'll call her for you."

"I will. I need to find one first though."

"Find one *what* first?" the fiancé asks. Are we playing "Who's on first"? What is going on?

"A doula!" I say again, exasperated.

"What do you mean? Don't you already know her?"

"Who?"

"Doula!"

"What? Oh my God," I say, cracking up. "Doula is not a person! Doula is what her job is called. You thought there was one woman out there named Doula who was a doula?"

"You mean doula is a job title and there's not a woman named Doula who helps during labor?" the fiancé asks, stunned.

"Exactly!"

"God, I'm an idiot," the fiancé says, embarrassed. "I really did think there was a woman named Doula."

"Yes, yes you are. Thanks for the laugh."

I haven't laughed so hard in what seems like years.

AUGUST 1

I just received an invitation for a baby shower in honor of Vivian and her husband, thrown by one of Vivian's old college friends, Stella. The gathering is set to take place at four o'clock next Sunday at Stella's house, located in a chic but suburban part of the city. In other words, a part of the city perfect for the young families who can afford to live there.

"Boy oh Boy!" reads the top of an invitation—everyone knows Vivian is having a boy—decorated with baby-bottle and rattle illustrations. Cute, I guess, if you're into that sort of thing.

I've never been to a baby shower before. Ronnie never had baby showers. She had parties for her babies after she gave birth. I made it to only one.

For one gathering I was too hungover to leave my house. The gathering for her second child was a breakfast thing and I slept through it. And I can't remember the last time I was invited to a party that started at four o'clock on a Sunday. Can anyone have fun at such a thing?

But it was for Vivian *and* her husband, which sounded more promising than baby showers where only women are invited. A women-only gathering is a waste of lipstick. I mean, what's so fun about spending the afternoon with a bunch of women oohing and ahhing over things for a baby, drinking tea and no alcohol? Not that I can drink anyway, even when there is a bar. I don't think I can even pretend to ooh and ahh at gifts. I don't think I have ever oohed and ahhed at anything, except maybe a photo of Brad Pitt topless. But at least there will be men there. And food. Perhaps even chocolate cake? If I'm going to a baby shower at four o'clock on a Sunday, there had better be chocolate cake. In any case, I will not be oohing and ahhing over anything. Not even for Vivian.

AUGUST 3

I met Sara for lunch today. We mostly talked about being pregnant.

"Are your ribs killing you?" Sara asked me, diving into her plate of fries.

"No, what do you mean?" I asked, diving into my plate of fries. Sara's portion looked larger than mine. Not fair!

"I swear I think my baby is legs up, pushing up against my ribcage. Or maybe it's the baby's ass. I'm not sure what it is, but something is pushing up against my ribs and it is incredibly painful. I've been jumping up and down for three days now trying to get it to move," she said.

"No, I don't have that pain. But I do get these weird cramps in my lower left side which last a couple days, kind of like period cramps."

"Yeah, I have those too."

"Those are a bitch."

"But those are nothing like this damn pain in my ribs," she moaned.

"You know I've had french fries every day now for six months?" I told her.

"Come on. Really?" she asked, rubbing her ribcage.

"Really. I'm not lying. I've had french fries every day for six months."

"Well, at least you're enjoying yourself."

"Yeah, you'd think so, right? But I'm not. French fries are an obsession now. It's scary, really."

Sara wasn't listening. She was too busy rubbing her ribs, with a pained expression on her face.

Later I call the fiancé. "Sara was telling me over lunch today that she has this bad pain in her ribs because of her baby. Maybe that's the one bad thing about pregnancy that I escaped."

"Well, that's good. Aren't you happy about that?"

"Yes, that's good."

"So what did you have to eat for lunch?"

"A big salad."

"Really?"

"Really."

"Really?"

"No."

"Fries?" he asks. Damn. The fiancé knows me too well.

AUGUST 4

"My ribs are killing me. They are killing me! I think I have what Sara has!" I cry to the fiancé.

"I'm going to kill Sara for telling you about her rib problems. You always manage to catch what everyone else has. She should know that about you," the fiancé says.

"Yeah. Me too," I moan.

God, my ribs are really killing me. Why does my baby *want* to hurt me so badly? What have I ever done to her?

AUGUST 5

10:00 p.m.

It was a beautiful evening. Cute Single Man and I went for a walk. I feel awkward about it now. Not because I'm technically really doing anything wrong—am I?—but because strangers look at him as if he's the father when we're out together. I can tell. They look at my stomach first, then they look at me, then at him. And then they smile—at *us.* "We're not together," I want to tell them. "There is no *us.*"

It is weird that I go out walking not with the father of my child but with another man. I know this. My relationship with Cute Single Man, if you can call it that, is not normal. Yet Cute Single Man is the only one who makes me forget about being pregnant, at least when people aren't smiling at us like we're happy parents-to-be. He makes me feel normal. Plus, he's *here,* unlike the fiancé, who is far, far away. A long-distance relationship used to seem like a good, novel idea, didn't it?

251

AUGUST 6

Had another appointment with Dr. G. this morning. While waiting to be called in, I realized that the waiting room of an obstetrician's office is much like a high school cafeteria—all of us pregnant chicks checking each other out. We give each other the once-over and we don't even try to hide it. We need to know what type of maternity clothes the others are wearing, to see who looks best, who is the more stylish pregnant woman. Does she look pregnant from behind? Does she look more or less worn down than I do? Has she gained more or less weight? Is her partner cute?

I noticed one or two envious looks directed my way. They certainly weren't inspired by my outfit (men's track pants, free promotional T-shirt for a coffee company) or by the size of my ass (colossal). The looks were directed at my new Prada bag. (Thanks for noticing!) When you are pregnant and you can't dress the way you like, the only thing you have left is to accessorize. It's okay to make yourself feel better by spending a ton of money on things you know you won't grow out of. And I now have a funky handbag to go with my funky mood and with the bags I already have— under my eyes.

As I was leaving, my phone rang.

"So how was the appointment?"

"It was good."

"So baby is good?"

"Yep."

"You're good?"

"I'm good. All is good."

"That's great. You rock!" said Cute Single Man, who had called before the fiancé.

It's just so wrong. He is not the father of this child, so why is he acting like the father? Why am I letting him act like the father? Maybe I need therapy.

I knew it. All my friends now want to be pregnant, even my "fun" friends.

"I just don't know when it's ever going to happen for me," Heather moans over the phone. "Charlie and I have been fighting like cats and dogs. I don't know if we have a future together."

"You have lots and lots of time to have a baby," I tell her. I didn't think someone as put-together as Heather ever worried about getting pregnant.

"But I want to be a young mother like you!"

"Trust me, it will happen."

"What if it doesn't work out with Charlie? What if nobody ever wants to have a baby with me?"

"Someone is going to want to have a baby with you. You have nothing to worry about."

"Okay, if I get pregnant within a year," Heather continues, "then our babies will basically be the same age, right?"

"Right."

"Then maybe by the time I get pregnant, you'll be on your second child and we can be pregnant together," she tells me. "Wouldn't that be great?"

Gaa!

"Let me get through this one first before we have me being pregnant again," I tell her, laughing.

Call me an evil person, but I'm going to hold off telling her how awful being pregnant is and let her envy me just a little bit longer. I know this feeling won't last. I'd better enjoy it while I can.

"Anyway, I've got to go," Heather tells me. "This magazine asked me to do a photo shoot and the stylist wants to meet me to dress me in some fabulous, slinky dress that I could never afford. They may even let me keep it. And then I have to go meet Charlie for drinks at this new bar downtown."

See? I knew the feeling wouldn't last.

AUGUST 9

Why am I so worried about giving birth? There are nearly six billion people in this world, and we each came out of a woman's body somehow. If six billion women can have a baby come out of them, so can I. But what if I'm the one pregnant woman who can't?

AUGUST 10

10:00 a.m.

Fuck! I forgot to buy Vivian a baby gift for her shower this afternoon. Could I use the pregnancy card—"Sorry! Didn't get you a gift because I've been too tired to leave the house"—or would that be rude? Of course that would be rude. What am I thinking?

Pregnancy can get you out of almost anything. It's come in handy when I visit my parents and want to leave immediately after dinner. It's gotten me out of work assignments that I don't find interesting. It's excused me when bailing out of plans, at the last minute even, when I realize I'm really not in the mood to go out. Pregnancy, if used correctly, is kind of like a Get Out of Jail Free card. But nothing excuses showing up giftless for your good friend's baby shower, especially pregnancy. It is pregnancy we're celebrating, after all.

1:00 p.m.

After dropping by a fancy kids' clothing store near my house and seeing that it was closed Sundays (don't they realize that baby showers usually occur Sunday afternoons and that there are a lot of people out there, like me, who leave buying gifts to the very last minute?), I race over to a nearby spa, which I've frequented and where I remember seeing Baby Spa items for sale. I purchase baby lotions, baby shampoos and conditioners, and fancy baby oils. I also pick up some pretty-smelling lotions for Vivian. Just because the shower is technically for her baby doesn't mean Vivian shouldn't receive gifts for herself. I mean, what has the baby done really, except be conceived? It's we pregnant women who have to do all the work. We not only deserve presents, we deserve medals.

4:45 p.m.

"Hi, I'm Stella. Welcome to my home. Come in! Everyone is out back. We were starting to worry that you guys had gotten lost, even though I had put the exact directions on the invite."

It is Shannon's fault we are late. She's never on time, even though I warned her it would be in bad form to show up late to a baby shower. Everyone else has already arrived. Apparently, baby showers are like weddings and funerals. If it's called for four o'clock, you are supposed to arrive at four o'clock.

"I think I remember meeting you about a year and a half ago," Stella says to me, as we walk through her kitchen. "We met at one of Vivian's Christmas parties, but I was very pregnant when we first met, so I'm not sure if you recognize me now. I remember thinking when we were introduced that you were so skinny. And now look at you! Now I'm skinny and you're big!" she continues, giving a little twirl to show off her toned, nearly anorexic body. "I lost all my weight *plus* another ten pounds. Can you believe I have two kids? You are really big. You sure you're not having twins?" she laughs. Ha ha. So funny. This party has started out fabulously.

"Hey, is there chocolate cake anywhere?" is the only response I can think of, aside from slapping skinny Stella on one of her bony cheekbones.

5:00 p.m.

It became clear as soon as I joined the gathering in Stella's backyard that there is a great divide between Vivian's friends. Half of the guests at her shower are parents, the other half non-parents. The parents stuck together, talking in small circles. The non-parents stuck to themselves as well. I didn't know any of the parents at the gathering.

At first I hung out with Lena, Shannon, Heather, and Marci—my non-mother friends. But then I started talking with some of the parents, who all asked me questions about my pregnancy, dishing out advice on how to get through the next couple of months. I am actually interested in what they had to say, even about their kids. What is *happening* to me? I'm not worried about boring these people with my pregnancy woes. It seems that once you've been pregnant, the topic of pregnancy *never* becomes boring. And once you have kids, talking about them *never* becomes boring either.

Heather, Shannon, Marci, and Lena are not getting the same kind of attention that I am. It feels kind of nice. I mean, you can't moan and make fun of heartburn and back fat unless you've been through it or are going through it. Unless you are or have been pregnant, you can't possibly understand what it's like. And you shouldn't even pretend to.

5:30 p.m.
"Oooohhh, that's so cute! Check out the little suspenders on those pants. Ahhh, I love it. I want that outfit for myself. Ooohhh, did you see the little ears on that stuffed rabbit? That is soooo

adorable. I can't get over how cute that stuffed animal is. Ahhh."

Gaa! Did that really come out of *my* mouth?

5:32 p.m.

"Ooohhh, look at those little running shoes. Could they *be* any cuter?" Eeek! Was that *me* again?

5:33 p.m.

"Vivian, open that present, over there, the one with the 'It's a Boy' ribbon on it. Is that what I think it is? No, it couldn't be. Oh, it is! It's a Winnie-the-Pooh doll! I love Winnie-the-Pooh. He's sooo cute . . . Oooohhh."

Ahh!!! It *is* me. Seriously, what is *happening* to me? I can't stop oohing and ahhing. I am a woman possessed.

6:30 p.m.

That was a fantastic shower. I wanted to stay longer, but Shannon wanted to leave. She had a date with her on-again-off-again boyfriend. It didn't matter. My voice was getting hoarse anyway, what with all the oohhing and ahhing. Vivian also received a Louis Vuitton diaper bag as a gift, which was much better than my Baby Spa items. How can you compete with a $1,400 Louis Vuitton diaper bag? I clearly need a friend who works at Louis Vuitton.

AUGUST 11

This pregnancy thing is hopeless. I can't cross my legs anymore when I sit down. I have to sit as though I was raised by wolves in a forest. My legs can't shut because my big belly gets in the way. I'm like a football player sitting on a bench. What next? Will I start spitting out tobacco?

AUGUST 12

I met Heather for an early dinner tonight, in an attempt to not hide from my old life.

"I'm sorry I'm late! I'm sorry, I'm sorry!" I yell out, racing into the restaurant, where Heather is waiting by the bar, nursing a beer. "I made the mistake of walking here and I have no concept of just how slow I walk these days."

"You're twenty minutes late! I was about to leave."

"Sorry! I'll pay for dinner. I swear, walking around with all this extra weight really slows me down. A blind man with a cane sped past me. That's how slow I'm walking these days."

"Well, you're here now. Do you want a drink? Oh, sorry, I guess you can't have an alcoholic drink, though I don't think one glass of wine will hurt you."

"No, I'm not going there. I still have caffeine and we're at a sushi restaurant. I can at least do

one thing right for this baby. I'll have a Perrier.
Can you believe the person I am now? I'm a former party girl on Perrier," I moan.

"You don't mind if I have another though, do
you?" Heather asks, turning to the bartender to
put in her order before I can answer. "I'm still a
party girl," she says.

Heather is a party girl on a diet, which is why she
wanted to go out for sushi. She's only eating
sashimi these days, for the protein-no-carbs
thing. It's a gloriously warm evening. We move to
the patio behind the restaurant. Is it just because
I'm pregnant, I think as we walk through the
restaurant, or is every woman here super skinny?

"You're looking so good," I tell Heather as we sit
down. She is. I have never seen Heather look slim-
mer. "And I'm getting fatter and fatter," I lament.

"Well, you are pregnant," she says. "That is what
happens when you get pregnant. I wish I could
have a picture of us together. This is the first time
ever that you are actually bigger than me. I need
proof that this is happening."

Why, oh why, did I ever agree to go out for dinner with Heather? "Don't worry," Heather says.
"The weight will come off eventually."

"Yeah, I'm giving myself two months after I give
birth to lose all the weight I've gained," I tell her.

"Two months? Are you crazy? You know what
they say, don't you? The general rule is nine
months to pack the pounds on, nine months to
get the pounds off."

"No, I can't have all this extra weight on for nine months. I'm giving myself two months and that's it."

"Not going to happen," Heather says, singsong-like.

"It is too. Wanna bet?"

"Seriously?"

"Yes, seriously. Let's make a bet. I bet that I will get back down to my pre-pregnancy weight by, let's say, December 31st. That will be two and a half months after the baby is born. Is that fair?"

"You're on. What should we bet? Dinner?"

"Dinner? No way," I scoff. "Dinner won't motivate me. I can afford to pay for my own dinner. We have to bet bigger than that. How about $250? Cash."

"Okay, $250 that you can't lose all that weight by New Year's."

"Are you willing to go higher? Like, let's say, $500?"

"Yes. Let's do $500."

I've given up alcohol. Apparently gambling's now my vice of choice.

"Okay. You're on. That will get me motivated for sure to lose the weight," I tell her.

"Hmmm," says Heather. "Whatever will I do with that easy extra $500 I will make off you?"

"Hey, Heather. Do you have any cigarettes on you?"

"Yeah, I have a couple. Why? Do you want one?"

"Yeah. You won't tell anyone, will you?"

"No. My mother smoked all during her pregnancy with me, and I've turned out just fine." I still have my secret stash of cigarettes hidden under my couch cushion. But, for fear of being stoned, I would never dare bring a pack of cigarettes out in public.

"Okay, but do I look pregnant right now?" I ask, moving my chair as close to the table as I can, trying to hide my big, pregnant belly underneath the tabletop.

"No, you can't tell you're pregnant when you push yourself under the table like that. You just look like you have really big breasts."

She hands me a cigarette and lights a match, and I inhale the first drag. It's nice to have friends who don't judge you.

"So are you walking back home?" Heather asks as we settle the bill.

"Are you crazy? If I walk home, I won't get there until tomorrow. I'll take a taxi."

Though if I plan to lose all my weight within two months after giving birth, I should probably walk. Fuck it, I think, waving down a cab. I'm pregnant.

AUGUST 14

I haven't been on the pill for a decade. I wasn't good on the pill. Meaning I would forget to take my birth control pills on a daily basis like you're supposed to. Then I would have to pop five pills in one night to make up for the forgotten pills, which doesn't work anyway, so I just went off it. Plus, I was on the pill while still living at home. I was always afraid my parents would find the stash and then they'd know that I was having sex.

"I'm going to go on the pill when this is done," I tell the fiancé during our nightly goodnight conversation. "They have this new kind of birth control which is like the patch and you just stick it on your back and it stays there all the time. I think you only have to change it once a month."

"Or I can get a vasectomy," the fiancé answers. Excuse me?

"You would do that?" I ask him, stunned. Aren't men fiercely protective of their private parts? Most men I know refuse to go to a doctor even when they're really ill. What kind of man offers to go in for the snip-snip?

"Maybe. We can discuss it later," he answers. Is the fiancé fearful that my way of birth control won't work and that we'll end up being pregnant again? Or is he just being kind?

AUGUST 16

The fiancé bought a house. Just like that. He called me, out of breath, to tell me about it.

"I can't believe I just did that. I put in the offer this morning and they just accepted it. The house has everything I want in a house. It's the most perfect location on a beautiful property. And it has everything you demanded in a house, too. It's within walking distance of a Starbucks. That's all you wanted, right?"

"I can't believe it," I told him. "That's amazing."

"I know. You're going to love it. It has four bedrooms and a huge kitchen and backyard. It needs a lot of renovation, but I already got the name of a good architect in town. There's just one little problem."

"What?"

"We can't move in until June. And depending on the renovations we want, we might not be able to move in for at least a year. Do you think we'll be okay with a baby for a while in my condo?" he asked.

"I always thought we'd be okay in your condo with a baby. In New York and Hong Kong, families of, like, eighteen live in tiny apartments."

Truthfully, I'm happy we won't have to move into a new house immediately. I'm still not entirely used to the idea that I will be living with the fiancé in his city, let alone living with him in a new city in a new home. Then again, I'm still not used to the idea that we're going to have a baby.

AUGUST 18

I have what will probably be my last appointment with Dr. G. this morning. I haven't figured out a way to tell him that he in fact won't be delivering my baby because I'm going to have her in the fiancé's city. It seems so wrong to have met with him all these times and then not have him see this "project" to the end. He's been so nice. It's almost like having to ditch a hairdresser you always enjoy talking to when you no longer like the way he cuts your hair. Hairdressers don't take too kindly to being dumped. Do obstetricians? I figure I'll ditch him by telephone, leaving a message on his office machine at midnight, when I can be sure no one is around to pick up the phone. I won't be the runaway bride, I'll be the runaway pregnant lady. I just hope his feelings won't be too hurt.

AUGUST 20

Shannon called. "That man I was seeing who went AWOL called me last night. He wants to get back together. I'm weak, I know. But I really like him. So I went over to his house and I think we're back on now."

"So you had make-up sex, right?"

"Yeah."

"And how was it?"

"It was fantastic. Unbelievable."

I'm now living vicariously through my girl-friends. I'm happy to report that at least someone out there is having sex, and the best kind too—make-up sex. Maybe I should start a fight with the fiancé? Maybe that will force me to have wicked sex again. The last time we had wicked sex was the night this child was conceived.

AUGUST 22

9:00 p.m.

My worlds have collided. Cute Single Man has just asked me if there is a sexy new intern working at my paper.

"Yes," I say, hesitantly. "Why?"

"Because one of my friends knows her and wants to set her up with me. Should I go?"

This. Cannot. Be. Happening. I am not ready to give up Cute Single Man. He's mine! Not that he's really mine. But I'm certainly not ready to give up Cute Single Man to Sexy Young Intern. This. Is. Not. Happening.

"Yeah. She's really hot," I tell him. "And talented too. She just wrote this great feature on trans fat and how awful it is for you." Why am I pimping for her? I want to tell Cute Single Man that no, under no circumstances is he allowed to meet her. But who am I, an engaged pregnant woman who is in love with her fiancé, to demand such a thing?

"So should I go?" he asks.

"Why not? You could have fun."

"Yeah, I guess I'll get her number and at least call her."

This. Cannot. Be. Happening.

"Would you mind if I called her?" Cute Single Man asks me.

"No, why would I mind? It's not like you're my boyfriend or anything," I spit out. Why did I have to spit that out? Why can't I remain calm and breezy?

"Are you sure?"

"Of course I'm sure. Listen, I have to go. I'm really tired. I want to go to sleep. I have a big day tomorrow. Lots of work." To keep up with Sexy Young Intern, who seems to be getting front-page stories every other day now.

Cute Single Man isn't attached. Neither is Sexy Young Intern. God, they have so much in common.

11:00 p.m.

I couldn't fall asleep. I had too many horrific thoughts going through my head about Cute Single Man getting married, living happily ever after. I couldn't help it. I got out of bed and called Cute Single Man back.

"I'm sorry for being grumpy and getting off the phone with you so suddenly. I'm just in a bad mood."

"Does your bad mood have anything to do with me telling you that I might call that intern at your paper?"

"Maybe a bit," I admit. "But most of it I think is hormones. I can't control them."

"If you tell me not to call her, I won't. Do you want me not to call her?"

"Yes. I want you not to call her."

"Really?"

"Really."

"Okay, I won't."

I blame my reaction on two things: One, I'm female. Females get jealous and insecure. Two, I'm pregnant. Together, the mix is toxic.

AUGUST 26

The fiancé has a lead on a nanny. It wasn't even a question whether we would get a nanny. I don't want to stop working entirely. How do women leave the workforce after working so hard to make their mark? What happens to all those years working their way up once they leave? How can women feel secure about what they've accomplished when there are younger, sexier, not-pregnant interns out there waiting to take over the world?

Of course, my baby only has her first year once and I don't really want to miss that. But doesn't hanging out with a baby all day long drive a woman wonky? Ronnie tells me stories about dying for adult company after days spent with her babies. "Sometimes it can be really hard," she once told me. "My husband will come home from work and want peace and quiet and I won't stop yapping at him. He doesn't understand what it's like to not have any grown-ups to talk to all day long. I find it hard sometimes to even form a sentence, I get so used to talking baby talk."

A nanny allows one to still have a life. Plus, a good nanny knows what she's doing, unlike the fiancé and me.

"She's supposedly excellent," says the fiancé. "She's worked with newborns before. My mother knows someone who knows her."

"So she's free to work for us?"

"She's prepared to leave her other job for us. Next time you're here, we'll meet her and see if we like her. Okay?"

"Okay. Is that allowed?"

"What?"

"Stealing someone's nanny."

"From what I understand," says the fiancé, "it's war when it comes to getting a good nanny."

"When is the next time I'm coming to visit you, anyway?"

"When would you like to come?"

"Well, I'm not sure how much longer I can fly. Some airlines say you're not allowed to fly past six months."

"That seems early to not be able to fly. Why is that?"

"I'm not sure. Maybe the airlines are scared pregnant women will go into labor or something and they'll have to make an emergency landing or call out on the speaker like in the movies, 'Is there a doctor on board? Is there a doctor on board?'

But it's only a four-hour flight to get to you. Even if I go into labor on the airplane, a baby won't pop out that quickly, right?"

"I guess. That would be a nightmare."

"We probably shouldn't leave it very much longer. I was thinking that maybe you'll come here and then we'll go back together, so you can help me bring all my stuff."

"Will you have a lot of stuff?"

"No, just clothes and my laptop. And I don't really have that many clothes left that fit me. How about the third weekend in September?"

"Sounds good to me."

"That's in like three weeks! In three weeks, we'll be living together."

"Yes, I know."

"Are you sure you still want me to move in with you?"

"Of course. You still want to be with me, right?" the fiancé asks.

"Of course! I love you."

Finally, after five years in this long-distance relationship, I'll be living with the fiancé. Then a few weeks later we'll have a baby. I wonder if we'll get along living under the same roof. God, we'd better get along. Or else we're screwed. I'm already making mental plans for the next time I can come back to visit my apartment, though. With the baby. Oh. My. God.

9:30 p.m.

Beep!

"Hi. This is Rebecca Eckler calling. I'm really sorry to have to tell you this, but I've decided to have my baby with the fiancé in his city. It's getting too hard to be here alone. But I want to thank you for everything. Once again, you won't be seeing me for any more appointments. But thanks for everything."

The Runaway Pregnant Lady just left a message for Dr. G. I am a coward. There was no way anyone would be picking up the phone on a Sunday night.

SEPTEMBER 1

I lost it on Cute Single Man tonight over a dairy product. We had plans that he'd come over, and I had asked him to stop along the way and pick me up a carton of chocolate ice cream. I was dying for ice cream. I didn't think I could live *one more second* without chocolate ice cream.

"Here," he said, handing me the plastic bag with the carton in it. I peeked inside the bag. Ahh, chocolate ice cream. Wait . . . that wasn't chocolate ice cream.

"What is this?" I asked him.

"Ice cream. Like you asked."

"No, I asked for *chocolate* ice cream and this is *toffee-flavored* ice cream. You have to go back to the store. You have to go back *now*."

"I'm not going back. Taste it. Trust me, it's amazing. It's so much better than chocolate."

"NO. I WANT CHOCOLATE ICE CREAM. GO BACK AND BUY CHOCOLATE ICE CREAM LIKE YOU SAID YOU WOULD."

"Trust me, you'll love this ice cream. I was trying to be nice."

"No you weren't! You bought the ice cream flavor *you* wanted, not the kind *I* wanted. I'll go get it myself then!" I screamed, throwing on my jacket. "AND YOU'D BETTER BE GONE WHEN I GET BACK."

He was gone when I got back. I think I crossed the line. I don't think I'll ever see him again. If anyone ever screamed at me like that—and over ice cream—I wouldn't ever want to see that person again either, even if she was pregnant. I'm a horrible, horrible person.

I tasted the toffee-flavored ice cream after he left. Cute Single Man was right. I loved it.

SEPTEMBER 2

"I'm really, really, really, really sorry," I tell Cute Single Man over the phone. "Will you please forgive me? I can't control my cravings. I can't control my emotions."

"What was that last night? I have never seen someone get that angry."

I was prepared to sob, if I had to, to get him to forgive me. "I am really sorry. I promise, it won't happen again."

"Okay, and I promise to get you chocolate ice cream next time. I don't want to see you like that ever again."

Even cute single men have their limits with pregnant women.

SEPTEMBER 3

My stomach feels like it's been attacked by hundreds of mosquitoes. It is so itchy, I can't stand it. Maybe I should put on oven mitts.

"Ronnie, you have to help me. My stomach is so itchy."

"Of course it is. That's what happens when the skin stretches out."

"But what do I do about it? I can't stop scratching, and it's not helping."

"There's nothing you can do about it really except lather on the coconut butter oil, or vitamin A and E oil—and thick."

ARGH. I head back to the washroom and butter myself up. Oiling myself up would be considered sexy—if I wasn't so pregnant.

I have decided Cute Single Man and I have to have a Talk. A Talk is something no woman looks forward to. Like when you have to ditch a man who is really nice and sweet but who you are not attracted to and who you realize you will never be attracted to, no matter how hard you try. Or when you want to know where the relationship with the man you are dating is going and have wanted to know where it's going for weeks and weeks but you are too shy to be the one to bring it up. Or a Talk can be just a result of insecurity and wanting to know that the guy you are dating is as into you as you are into him.

The Talk I need to have with Cute Single Man is different from any other Talk I've ever had before. How do I go about ending something when there's nothing concrete to end? I have decided that after the ice cream meltdown, I can't continue with him. It's too weird. It's too . . . nice. I have not fallen in love with Cute Single Man. But somehow over the past couple of months, I have fallen deep in *like* with Cute Single Man. It has to end. I do not want to screw things up with the fiancé, whom I love to pieces. I will call Cute Single Man and ask him to come over tomorrow. I will tell him that "we have to talk," so he'll be braced for what's to come. Everyone, after all, knows what the "We have to talk" line leads to.

8:00 p.m.

"So what is it we need to talk about?" Cute Single Man asks, plopping himself down on my couch, moving into a far corner so there is room for me to plop down beside him. "You sounded serious."

"Um, this is hard. What is it we're doing here?"

"What do you mean?"

"Don't you find this all a little strange? I'm starting to get weirded out."

"About us?"

"Yes, about us. I can't do this anymore. I got jealous when you mentioned you were going to call that intern at my paper. I'm not supposed to be jealous. I'm engaged! I love my fiancé! I'm going to have a baby in two months! So what is it we're doing?"

"I don't know. But aside from the ice cream argument, I'm enjoying myself. Aren't you?"

"Well, yeah. But I can't. I don't think we should see each other anymore. And I don't think we should talk anymore. I need to focus on my baby and my future, and I can't handle any more stress, and whatever it is we're doing is stressing me out. I'm moving cities soon and moving in with my fiancé. I'm going to have a *baby*, in case you haven't noticed."

Cute Single Man is silent.

"So, um, what do you think?" I say, pressing him. I feel dizzy.

"I know. This is fucked. Are you sure you don't want to see me anymore? Are you sure this is what you want?"

"No, I'm not sure about anything. But I can't do this, whatever it is we're doing. I just can't."

"If this is what you want, then I'll respect your decision."

"I really like you," I tell Cute Single Man. "I might like you too much, and that's the main problem. If we don't end whatever it is we're doing now, what am I going to do when I live in a different city? I rely on you too much."

"I know what you mean. I'm going to miss you."

"I'm going to miss you too."

"I'm going to miss Baby too. I guess there's nothing else to say, then. I guess I should split."

"Well, you don't have to leave right away. You can stay a bit, can't you?" Don't go! Don't go!

"No, I think it's best if I leave now. I'm sad now. Can I get a hug before I leave?" he says.

"Yes," I say. We hug and look into each other's eyes the way people do before they are about to kiss for the first time. Is he going to? If it's going to happen, it's going to happen now. Will I kiss back? But Cute Single Man pulls away quickly, gives my belly a soft pat, and walks out my door, shutting it loudly behind him.

My heart pounds and I feel out of breath. I feel like I've just been dumped. How am I going to get through this when, technically, there is nothing to get through?

1:00 a.m.

Cute Single Man has not called. Why hasn't he called? Isn't he missing me at all? Did I make a mistake? Why couldn't we just be friends? Should I call him? I can't. I just can't. We are not talking anymore. I was the one who ended it, and now I have to live with it.

SEPTEMBER 7

I need to call Cute Single Man. Everyone always told me to never get your hair cut when you're pregnant because you're not thinking clearly and don't want to make any rash decisions. It doesn't happen as often, but maybe you shouldn't end a relationship or a friendship during pregnancy either. Was I too rash? Pretty soon I'll be in another city anyway, so what does it matter if we continue to hang out until then? No. I can't call. I just can't.

SEPTEMBER 8

AHHHH!!! My belly button is missing. MY BELLY BUTTON IS MISSING! Where did it go? It's just . . . disappeared. It's vanished. My belly button, apparently, has been so stretched out it's completely gone. What if it doesn't come back? What if I never see my belly button again?

I wonder if there's a plastic surgeon out there who can do reconstructive surgery on a belly button. I miss my belly button. I miss Cute Single Man.

SEPTEMBER 9

Vivian, who has worn her pregnancy as well as Sarah Jessica Parker wears Dolce and Gabbana, is in a foul mood. I am too. It's been two days since I've heard from Cute Single Man. I miss him. And I can't talk to any of my girlfriends about it, the way we always do when one of us goes through a breakup. But I've never seen Vivian in a sour mood. She's usually so happy. But, boy, is she sour now.

"My doctor told me five days ago that it could happen anytime now. I've been waiting five days and nothing. Not one damn contraction. I've been running around like crazy these past few days getting everything ready, and now everything is ready, and we still don't have a baby. I want to have this baby out of me. Now!" she grumbles.

"Have you tried spicy food?" I ask her.

"Why?"

"Haven't you heard that spicy food is supposed to bring on labor? Everyone knows that. Maybe you should drink a bottle of Tabasco sauce or something."

"Well, I have been eating Indian food and I'm still pregnant!"

"How about sex? I heard that sex also induces labor. Maybe you and your hubby should do it."

"We just had sex two nights ago and that didn't work."

Phew. I was happy to learn that Vivian couldn't handle the idea of sex anymore either. I can't even remember when the fiancé and I last had sex, and if you can't remember, that's not a good sign.

"Well, I think you have to do it two times in a row for it to work," I tell her.

"Maybe I'll try Indian food again tonight. I can't have sex again. It's too uncomfortable."

"Okay, no sex. But how about walking? Have you walked briskly?"

"Yes. I went on three brisk walks yesterday and nothing, nothing, nothing!" Vivian is getting more upset with each suggestion.

"Calm down. Calm down," I tell her. "I also heard that Chinese food works."

"Chinese food? We've had Chinese food three times this week!"

"Yeah, you're right. Brisk walks, sex, spicy food, Chinese food—I'm sorry, but I guess they're all myths."

"Yeah, whoever made those things up are big, fat liars," Vivian moans.

"Maybe you should try eating Mediterranean food. Have a falafel or something."

"Why?"

"Why not? You never know, right?"

SEPTEMBER 10

Something truly distressing happened today. The weather turned chilly, which wouldn't normally be a disaster. That is what happens when summer ends. As North Americans, we know colder weather is always just around the corner. But I've realized that I can't bend over anymore, and that is a problem when it's too chilly to wear sandals and I can no longer bend down to put on socks. After five minutes I managed to get the socks on—albeit kind of twisted—by sitting on my bed, taking a deep breath, and lifting my leg into the air. The procedure took five minutes. Pregnancy is not only a pain in the ass, it's time consuming. I miss the old me, the one who could put on socks.

SEPTEMBER 11

Not being able to dress my own feet in socks was distressing. Then this morning in the shower I realized I can't wash my legs anymore. I can't bend down to lather them up with soap. Which means there is no way in hell I can reach to wash my feet, either. How long before they start to smell? God forbid I should drop the soap in the shower. Perhaps I should have a backup bar of soap in the shower with me from now on?

9:00 a.m.

I can barely wipe myself after I pee. My stomach is too large. No one—absolutely no one—warned me about this! The fiancé is arriving early tomorrow morning. I haven't packed a thing. And, even worse, my friends are making me go out to a media party tonight at a local television station. What the hell am I going to wear?

"Come on. You have to come out," demands Shannon. "You can wear whatever. Everyone is going. You can't hibernate just because you're pregnant. I haven't been to a good party in what seems like forever. Actually, the last good party I was at was the Conception Party."

"The what party? When was that?" Was there a good party I missed?

"Your engagement party in January! That's what we've all started to call it. The Conception Party," she tells me.

"Who's calling it that?"

"Everybody is calling it that. That's what it was, wasn't it?"

Oh. My. God.

What if I run into Cute Single Man? Maybe I want to run into Cute Single Man?

"You'll have fun. I promise. Pregnant women do have fun, you know."

"Shannon?"

"Yes."

"Please don't call my engagement party the Conception Party again."

11:00 p.m.

Going to the party was a huge mistake. I should never have left my apartment.

I looked as good as I could look, being eight months pregnant. I wore a low-cut black dress that showed off my pregnant cleavage, and knee-high red boots, which I shoved my pregnant feet into. I wanted to look good in case Cute Single Man was there. After any kind of breakup—even this strange one—it's always important to try to look your best when running into the ex. It's kind of like pay-back, in the see-what-you're-missing kind of way. Every woman knows that.

I first met Marci, Shannon, and a couple of others at a bar before heading over to the party. I sat watching them drink martinis while I nursed a cranberry and soda. Then we headed over to the party. Our names were checked off on the guest list and we headed into the mess of a few hundred people. I didn't see Cute Single Man anywhere.

"I really have to find a washroom," I told my friends. My bladder felt like it was going to explode. It had, after all, been fifteen minutes since I had last peed. "It's so packed in here. How am I going to find you guys?" I asked, sure that one of them would offer to come with me.

"We'll be right here. Don't worry. You'll find us, or we'll find you."

Working my way through the crowd was next to impossible. People were jammed together like sardines. I wanted to scream out, "PREGNANT LADY COMING THROUGH! PREGNANT LADY COMING THROUGH!" Of course, I didn't. I didn't want anyone to pay attention to me, I felt so out of place with my big belly. It took twenty minutes to find the washroom. When I got there, the line went out the doors. I was too embarrassed to push my way through saying, "I'm pregnant. I have to pee *now* or I'm going to have an accident." No one in this stylish, mostly tipsy crowd would understand what it's like to be pregnant. Plus they were all well on their way to getting drunk, so they probably had to pee as badly as I did. In addition to wheelchair-accessible washrooms, there should be special facilities for pregnant ladies.

I decided to leave immediately. There was no way I was going back through the crowd to find my friends, especially after running into a few acquaintances on the way to the washroom who told me that I looked "sexy . . . for a pregnant woman." I flagged down a taxi, and just as I thought I had surely drowned my baby in pee, I made it through my apartment door.

I called the fiancé in tears.

"Calm down. I'll be there tomorrow and we'll do something fun."

"Am I overreacting? Am I? Am I? Am I?" I now have to check with someone else to see if I'm overreacting. I know enough now to know to not always trust how I'm feeling. Pregnant hormones are a bitch.

"They probably just didn't know how badly you had to go," the fiancé said calmly.

"Well, I don't care if I'm overreacting. I'm never coming out of my apartment again."

I didn't even get to see Cute Single Man.

12:30 a.m.

Is that my phone? Who could be calling me at this hour?

"Hey, it's me." It's Cute Single Man. It's Cute Single Man!

"Oh . . . hey!" I'm suddenly awake.

"Did I see you tonight? I thought I saw you at a party, but it was too crowded to get to you."

"Yeah, I did go to a party. How are you?"

"Good. You looked good," he says.

"I felt like shit. I left ten minutes after getting there."

"Well, you looked good. I've missed you."

"I've missed you too. I'm moving in a few days."

"Really? That soon?"

"Yeah."

"Well, I just wanted to say hi. Good luck with everything, okay? And keep in touch, will you? I want to know how everything goes."

"Really?"

"Yeah, really. I feel like I've been there from the beginning and I want to know how it ends."

"Okay, I will."

"You promise?"

"Yeah, I promise."

"Promise again."

"I promise."

Tomorrow I start my life with the fiancé. No sense in being mean to Cute Single Man now.

SEPTEMBER 13

The fiancé has arrived. I'm so relieved he's here. When he's with me, everything seems better. Everything is better when he's around. The clock is ticking away, however. If we don't get shopping, our baby will be sleeping in the bathtub or on the floor or in the hallway, or worse—in *our* bedroom on *our* bed. The fiancé and I figured it would be easiest to get everything here and then get it shipped to his place. We're all about minimum effort. I, however, have to come out of my apartment.

"If the Pottery Barn was good enough for Vivian's baby room, it will be good enough for us," I tell the fiancé. "Do you know that Vivian has binders with sticky notes, and has cross-referenced all her research about cribs and change tables? She's already done the research for us."

"Let's make this quick and painless," I tell the fiancé, as he opened the heavy doors at the Pottery Barn for me.

"Yes, quick and painless."

"Let's not spend more than one hour in here. We need a deadline so we don't dawdle. Quick and painless."

"I'm with you."

"What's your watch at?" I ask him. "I have 1:30."

"Me too."

"So, we're out of here by 2:30, right?"

"Right. Quick and painless."

"So what do we do now?"

"Well, first, I suppose, we find out where the baby stuff is."

"Hey, do you like this coffee table?"

"Beck . . ."

"Right. I have to keep focused. Oh, there's a sign that says 'Baby' upstairs. Let's go. Fuck, please tell me there's an elevator. Screw it. I'll take the stairs. I can consider it my cardio for the last four months."

It's amazing how difficult climbing stairs has become. I hate to admit it, but I am huffing and puffing after climbing, I think, six stairs. (Is it really only six stairs?)

On the top landing, I take in the scene.

"Okay, now what?" I ask the fiancé.

"We buy stuff."

"Right. Ready, set, go. Wait . . . How do we know what we need exactly?"

"I guess we should have thought about that before we came. I see some cribs over there."

"I see something even better."

"Beck. We need a crib. Keep focused."

"No, what I mean is that I see a saleslady over there. We clearly need help."

"Good idea."

I chase down one of the salesladies. Bingo! She's pregnant. What could be more perfect than a pregnant saleslady in the Baby section of the Pottery Barn?

"Hi. Um, we're having a baby," I tell her, rubbing my stomach. "In, like, a month. We need a baby room. Can you help us?"

"Sure. Why don't we walk over to the crib section. We have a few different styles." I feel as though we are walking into the pages of a catalogue. This is going to be easy.

"Hey, look at this one," I tell the fiancé. "It's deep burgundy, the same color as the rest of your condo. It's perfect."

"Yep. I like it. We'll take it."

Fifty-four minutes to go.

"We'll take this, too," I tell the saleslady. "This is a change table, right? We need this, correct?"

"Correct," she responds.

"Do you know what else we need?" I ask.

"You'll need sheets, and blankets, and maybe a few of these wicker baskets to keep things organized. Do you know if it's a boy or girl?"

Fifty minutes and counting.

"We're having a girl."

"Well, we have sheets in blue and pink and yellow."

"Pink is good," I say, taking control. "We'll even take the mobile hanging over the crib. And we'll take some of those baskets you were talking about. And maybe this stuffed animal," I continue, picking up a lamb, which when you wind up its tail plays, I think, "Twinkle, Twinkle Little Star."

The saleslady starts packing everything up for us. The fiancé, at this point, is sitting in a chair talking to a friend on his cellphone.

"What other crap do we need?" I ask the saleslady.

"Crap?"

"Well, you know what I mean."

Forty-two minutes and counting.

She rings up all our purchases, including a breastfeeding pillow that wraps around your stomach and that the baby can lie on (in case I decide to breastfeed), a huge stuffed bear, and some wicker baskets for storage. She writes down the fiancé's address, and the fiancé hands over his credit card. The cost? $3,200.

"That wasn't so bad," I say to the fiancé as we walk out onto the street. "But who knew a baby room could be so expensive."

"That's what happens when you don't comparative shop," he answers.

The last thing you want to do when you're eight months pregnant is to spend your day comparative shopping. Who has the energy? Besides, the fiancé and I are too pleased with ourselves to worry about money right now. We just purchased an entire baby room in exactly twenty-eight minutes.

SEPTEMBER 14

Vivian had her baby! A boy, weighing 8 pounds, 3 ounces. I want to call her, but I know that you should always give a new mother a couple of days to recuperate. Ronnie told me that. I can't wait to talk to Vivian. I want to know everything. I send flowers to the hospital.

SEPTEMBER 15

I spend the day cleaning my apartment while the fiancé visits friends. I am going to be moving to his city in three days, and I have this over-whelming need to get my apartment in tip-top shape before leaving. I want my apartment to sparkle when I come back with the baby for visits. I must clean. I must clean. I must clean.

I clean under my washroom sink. I throw out three garbage bags of old clothes. I even empty my freezer (how long has that tub of ice cream been in there?) and my refrigerator (how did that leftover soup get in there?). This is a feeling I've never experienced before. I'm the type of gal that leaves used butter knives on the counter. I'm the type of gal that always leaves the cap off the toothpaste. I'm the type of gal that has no idea how to mop a floor or how to get fingerprints off walls. Is this the nesting instinct that I hear hits women right before their babies arrive?

The phone rings while I'm on the floor in my closet organizing my shoes. I don't make it to the phone. (Help! I've fallen and I can't get up!) I have to roll on my side, grab the lower rack in my closet, and pull myself up. It isn't pretty. I'm glad no one is around to see it.

SEPTEMBER 16

Remind me to never, ever give advice to anyone who tells me she is pregnant. Absolutely everyone in the world has advice to give you when you're pregnant. I realized that today after going for what should have been a relaxing hair appointment.

You want your haircut experience to be relaxing, especially after paying way too much money to get half an inch chopped off. But even my gay head-to-toe-Prada-wearing male hairstylist who loves-loves-loves plastic surgery couldn't help but throw in his two cents (which, in the high-priced-hairstylist world, is more like throwing in his $150).

"You are going to breastfeed, aren't you?" he asks, combing out my dripping wet hair.

Did my gay, Prada-wearing hairdresser really just ask me about breastfeeding? What next?

"Hmmm," I answer, nonchalantly.

The fiancé and I are leaning toward not breastfeeding. I know, we should be hanged.

"You absolutely must breastfeed, m'dear," he says.

"Um, you don't even have breasts. How do you know so much about breastfeeding?" I ask him.

"I have lots of clients who have had babies. They all say it is just a fabulous experience and so much better for the baby. Breastfeeding is fab-u-lous!"

"I was thinking about getting bangs," I tell him, trying to get him off the subject.

"I think bangs would be fabulous. Would make you a yummy mummy indeedy," he says.

"But maybe I should wait until after I have the baby. You're not supposed to make any rash decisions when you're pregnant, right?"

I wouldn't be able to handle it if I got a new hairstyle that made me look even uglier than I already feel. Plus, my face is now rounder than it's ever been. I now have what they call, if they're being nice, cherub cheeks. In fact, the last time I visited my grandfather, he actually pinched them, something he hasn't done since I was; oh, six.

"Okay, let's wait on the bangs then. Book an appointment after you give birth. You can even breastfeed while I cut! Won't that be fab-u-lous?"

"Oh yuck!" I respond.

"Don't be surprised," my hairdresser says, snipping away, "if some—or a lot—of your hair falls out after you give birth. It happens to a ton of women."

Gaa! I'm going to be bald, at age thirty!

I go to visit Vivian and her baby boy, David. It's unbelievable. Not so much the baby, but Vivian. Vivian, who gave birth five days ago, looks like she's lost almost all the weight she gained during pregnancy. She's like a freak of nature. I hate her.

"Are you wearing new jeans?"

"No, these are my old jeans," Vivian answers.

As soon as I walk into her kitchen Vivian says, "I hate to do this to you, but the nurses at the hospital were adamant that everyone who comes to visit David has to wash their hands before touching him."

She directs me to the sink, where a new bottle of antibacterial soap waits to be used, apparently, by all visitors. I can handle being told to wash my hands, but Vivian had better not check under my fingernails.

"So where's the little midget?" I ask.

"He's right there," she says, pointing to a corner of the kitchen where baby David is sleeping soundly in his car seat.

"Oh my God. I didn't even know he was there."

"I know. He's super quiet. He's a really great baby. All he does is sleep."

Vivian picks up David, and we move to her couch in the living room.

"Do you want to hold him?" she asks.

Suddenly I feel faint. I have never held a newborn before. "Um, maybe in a bit. Maybe I'll just watch him for a while first. Wow. It's really strange, isn't it? Watching him is like watching a reality TV show. But this is even better. It's really reality. Do you just sit here and stare at him all day?"

"Pretty much that's exactly what I do," Vivian answers. "Who do you think he looks like?"

"I'm not sure. He looks like a baby," I answer, not sure what the right answer is.

David is an adorable baby, which is good, because I understand that not all newborns are, especially when they have to come out the birth canal, which isn't big. Many babies have pimples, bruises, and bashed-in heads for the first week of their lives—though even I know you could never describe a baby as anything other than cute to a new mother.

"Um, maybe I'll try holding him now," I say, silently praying that David won't start to cry upon being put in my arms. That would make me feel really bad.

Vivian plops David into my arms. I know to hold up his head, at least. David just fits in the nook of my arm. I can feel the nervous sweat forming under my arms. Please don't cry, Baby David. Please don't cry.

"Hey, this isn't so bad. It's not bad at all," I say. "I was worried that I'd break him or something."

"I know. Babies are really more durable than you think."

Vivian's doorbell rings. She gets up to answer it.

"You're not leaving me alone with him, are you?"

"I'll only be gone a second," she says.

"But what if he starts crying?"

"I'm only going to be gone a second!"

It's one of her friends, Helen, whom I have met, briefly, a number of times before.

"Hey, I understand you're moving?" Helen says to me. I have just handed Baby David back to Vivian. I have had enough. Will I get tired of holding my own baby after ten minutes?

"Yep. I'm still keeping a place here, so I'm not moving entirely. It will keep our relationship strong, you know, to not always be together," I tell Helen.

"Yeah, that's the way to go. You never should spend that much time with your partner. You have to have him miss you a little."

I don't want to think about moving in with the fiancé right now. Not while five-day-old Baby David is in the same room, with no idea about how complicated his life will be when he meets a woman.

"Thanks for letting me hold him," I call out as I walk out Vivian's front door. "You know, that was the first time I've ever held a baby."

"What? It was?" she says, shocked.

"Yeah. I guess maybe I should have told you that before I held him."

No worries. I didn't break her baby. Thank God, I didn't break her baby.

I cry on the plane with the fiancé sitting next to me. There is nothing worse than not being able to control your tears in public. Thank God I have a window seat and can hide my face.

Before the plane took off, while we were waiting on the runway, it hit me. My life, as I have known it, is now over. At least for the foreseeable future, I'm leaving my friends, my family, my job. I will be living with the fiancé. I will be a mother. I am now, officially, forced to be a grown-up. I miss Cute Single Man.

The fiancé tries to calm me down by offering me a package of peanut M&M's. He knows I'm not entirely ready for all this change. The candy helps. I stop crying on the outside. Inside I am a mess.

My mother calls to see if I have arrived.

"So the airplane seatbelt fit over your stomach?" she asks. I might be big, but I am not four hundred pounds, for God's sake.

SEPTEMBER 19

9:30 a.m.

Maybe living here won't be that bad. The fiancé has strawberry jam in his fridge. I discovered it when I woke up.

Lena told me the other day that one of her friends ate a loaf of bread every morning during the last two months of her pregnancy. I didn't think it was possible for anyone—not even a professional wrestler—to eat an entire loaf of bread. How many slices of bread are in a loaf? Thirty? That is, I didn't think it was possible for anyone to eat an entire loaf of bread until I ate an entire package of English muffins this morning. It was all because of the strawberry jam.

The fiancé does not live within walking distance of a McDonald's, and he made it clear the minute we got off the plane that I would not be allowed to eat Big Macs in his company.

"Not on my watch," he answered when I asked if we could stop at the Golden Arches on the way to his place.

"But there's one right near here!" I protested.

"Not on my watch," he repeated.

I was annoyed, but I had already cried on the plane. A fight over a high-calorie sandwich wasn't worth it. It was clear, however, that I would need a new craving. So this morning I toasted an English muffin, buttered it thick, and topped it off with the strawberry jam I found. I ate it in twelve seconds. I needed another one. So I toasted another English muffin, buttered it, and spread on the strawberry jam. I did this five times before I stopped. Not because I was full, but because I had finished the package.

6:30 p.m.

The fiancé came home from work. He found me in bed, where I was lying watching bad television.

"Why do you look so sheepish?" he asked, coming over to kiss me.

"I don't know. This is the way I look."

"What have you done? I can tell you've done something. You have that look on your face."

"No, I'm just watching reruns of *Who's the Boss,* I swear! What are you doing?" I asked, mortified, watching as he unbuttoned his shirt.

"I'm coming into bed with you."

"Okay, but—" And before I could stop him, he jumped into bed. CRUNCH! CRUNCH! CRUNCH!

"What the fuck? What was that?" the fiancé yelled, whipping back the covers. "Oh my God, Beck," he said, starting to laugh. "I really can't believe you were hiding those under the covers."

The fiancé had landed on the super-size bag of Cheesies I had tried to hide under the covers when I heard him come in the door.

10:00 p.m.

My belly now moves on its own. Each night, as soon as I settle into bed, I watch my stomach. It moves *on its own.*

"What part of the body do you think this is?" I ask the fiancé, placing his hand on what I think is the baby's elbow sticking out.

"I have no idea. Maybe it's the leg?"

"I thought the baby was positioned the other way."

"No, it's positioned this way."

"Really?"

After all these months, I have no idea how my baby is positioned. Some women can tell exactly what part of their baby's body is sticking out. I cannot.

"Hand me that magazine over there," I tell the fiancé. I take the latest issue of *Us Weekly,* which was lying on the floor, and rip out a photo of Tom Cruise.

"Now watch this," I tell the fiancé, placing the page on my stomach. Tom Cruise's face moves up and down on top of my stomach. "Isn't that a neat little trick?"

"How weird."

"I know. And feel how hard my stomach is up here," I say, again taking the fiancé's hand and placing it this time right under my ribcage, where my stomach is as hard as a rock. "Why do you think it's so hard?" Each night, my stomach becomes super hard.

"I think that's her ass," the fiancé says.

"Yeah. Not even born yet and the baby already has a great butt."

SEPTEMBER 20

1:30 a.m.

I'm lying half on my stomach, with a pillow in between my legs. Note to self: Ask Dr. Bono at my next checkup if it's possible that I'm squishing my baby's brain by sleeping this way.

SEPTEMBER 21

7:00 a.m.

"Pancakes! Pancakes! Get out of bed, sleepy head. Me want pancakes! Pancakes!"

"Jesus, Beck. What time is it?"

"Pancake time!"

"Dear God."

"Let's go to Phil's. Please?" Phil's is a truck-stop diner.

"Can I shower first?"

"No time for showers. I need pancakes now! Pancakes! Pancakes!"

"All right. All right. Give me a second."

4:00 p.m.

One of the games I love playing with the fiancé is the "What if?" game. The fiancé hates this game, which I can understand—What if I gained 250 pounds? Would you still love me? What if you won 3 million dollars? How much would you give me? What if I died in a car accident? Would you be sad?—but he's being super patient because I'm super pregnant.

"What if my water breaks in your car and I ruin your leather seats? Would you be mad?"

"No, of course not."

"What if my water breaks on your couch and ruins it and you have to buy another one? Would you be mad?"

"No."

"What if my water breaks and you are out playing golf and I can't get in touch with you and you miss the labor?"

"That would never happen."

"But what if it does?"

"I promise to always carry my cellphone with me, even on the golf course. Whenever your number comes up on call display, I'll answer it."

"What if labor comes on really fast and you have to deliver the baby yourself because we don't have time to make it to the hospital and we're stuck in traffic?"

"That better not happen."

"But what if it does?"

"What if we stop playing this stupid 'What if?' game?"

"Fine."

2:00 a.m.

"I'm worried," I say to the fiancé.

"I'm tired."

"Really, I'm really, really worried."

"I'm really, really tired. What are you worried about now? About being a mother?"

"No. I mean, yes. But I'm not worried about that right now. I'm worried about going into labor early. I have no idea what to do if that happens. Do you?"

"No," the fiancé answers. "I guess we head to the hospital."

"I know that. But where do you go when you get to the hospital? Do you go to emergency, or are you supposed to go to a specific floor, like the maternity floor, or are you supposed to call your doctor as soon as you get your first contraction, like in the movies, and say, 'The baby is coming. Meet me at the hospital.' Or what?"

"I'm not sure. But you have a doctor's appointment tomorrow. We'll ask the doctor."

"And we don't even know what we're supposed to bring to the hospital. Do we have to bring something for the baby to wear right after she's born? Do we have to bring baby bottles if we're not breast-feeding? Do we have to bring diapers, and is someone going to teach us how to put on a diaper?"

"Beck, we'll ask the doctor tomorrow. Let's just try to get some sleep."

"Okay, but don't yell at me if I go into labor tonight and ruin your fancy sheets when my water breaks."

"Okay," he mumbles.

"Hey, what if that happened? Would you be mad?"

"What if you let me get some sleep?"

SEPTEMBER 23

8:00 a.m.

In Dr. Bono's examining room, the nurse greets me with the nine words no woman wants to hear at eight in the morning. "You have to get a Pap smear done today," she tells me.

"I do?" I say, turning to look at the fiancé. "Okay, you're going to have to leave the room for this."

"Yeah, you're right, I definitely must leave the room." The fiancé looks disgusted, but then again, so do I. No woman should be forced to have a sudden Pap smear. I need warning for something like that.

"Why do I need a Pap smear today?" I ask the nurse.

"It's to make sure you don't have any viruses that can be harmful to the baby when it's born," she explains. "But wait . . . You were thinking about having a C-section, right, last time you were here? If you have a C-section, you won't have to do this test."

I am so not in the mood to have a Pap smear. I would have to undress, get into a gown, and spread my legs for strangers and pretend that getting one done isn't so bad. There is nothing worse than a doctor trying to involve you in small talk while you are getting a Pap smear done. I am supremely tired and borderline grumpy already.

"Yes, yes I am. I am having a C-section," I say, turning to look at the fiancé.

"Great. Then we can forget about this test. The doctor will be in in one sec to see you," the nurse says, leaving the room.

"So, I guess you've decided to have a C-section then?" the fiancé asks.

"Looks that way. Do you think that's the right way to go?"

"It's totally up to you."

"But if you were a woman and you had to have a baby come out of you, would you do it?"

"Without a doubt, I'd get the C-section. But I can't believe you've decided to do the C-section because you're too lazy to get out of your clothes. That's the reason, isn't it?"

"Well, it's cold in here," I moan to the fiancé. "But that's not the real reason. I think you're right. In this day and age, I'd be crazy not to get one done. It really is so much easier. And I can't handle this waiting anymore. I want to know when I'm going to have my baby, and I want to know now."

Dr. Bono enters the room. "Hidee-ho! I understand you've finally made a decision? I'm a little surprised. Last time I saw you, you seemed to still be thinking about going the vaginal route."

"Well, I am female, after all. It's my prerogative to change my mind," I joke. "But now that my mind is finally made up, what day would you do the C-section?"

"Let's see," Dr. Bono says, looking at my chart and then looking at a calendar posted on the wall. "You're due around October 20th. I usually perform them on Wednesdays, so how is October 15th for you?"

"Um, I'll have to check my Palm Pilot," I joke again. "No, I'm kidding. I think I'm free. And what time would you do it?"

"How's 9 a.m.?"

"So, my baby will be born October 15th at 9 a.m.? Sounds good to me. Now this is a crazy thought, but what if I happen to go into early labor? What happens then?"

"You go to the hospital and tell them you had a scheduled C-section booked, and they should still be able to accommodate you."

"Perfect."

"And how long will she have to be in the hospital?" the fiancé asks.

"For C-sections, we like patients to stay three days."

"Three days? Do they have showers in the room?" I ask Dr. Bono.

"Of course they have showers."

"Well, how am I supposed to know? And how

long exactly will the scar be? And you'll do it low, right? So I can still wear a bikini?"

"The scar will be right over your pubic hairs. And it will be about six inches long. So I'll see you next week then?"

We now have weekly visits to Dr. Bono.

And that's that. I suddenly know my baby's birthday. On the way out, Dr. Bono's secretary hands us a sheet of paper that lists all the things we need to bring to the hospital. One of the items is maxi pads. Why do I need maxi pads if it's coming out of my stomach? I thought no bleeding Down There was one of the advantages of not going the vaginal route. But I'm not going to question it. I guess I'll buy some maxi pads. I haven't bought maxi pads in years.

"Hey, what are you thinking about? You kind of blanked out there for a minute," the fiancé says, waving his hand in front of my eyes.

"Nothing. Just the baby." I am not going to tell the fiancé that I was worrying about maxi pads. "Can you believe that we know exactly when we're going to have a baby?" I ask him while we wait for the elevator.

"I know. It's crazy. Does that make her a Scorpio?" What? I had no idea the fiancé even knew about signs, let alone cared about them. It's typically such a girlie thing.

"Actually, I think it means she will be a Libra."

"What are the traits of a Libra then?"

"I think Libras are wishy-washy. I think

Scorpios are more sane, but I'm not sure. Let's get a book on signs."

"Maybe we should think about getting some books on parenting instead. I'm not sure it matters what sign the child is when we don't know how to feed her."

"Yeah, maybe. But you're the one who brought up signs. We could get both. Maybe we should go back and ask Dr. Bono to move the C-section a couple weeks later so we can have a Scorpio child."

"Beck, no. Definitely not."

We make a pact to tell only our parents about the C-section.

4:00 p.m.

Lena just called. She told me she booked a two-week trip to New York. "There are a ton of good parties going on there now. And a bunch of new restaurants I want to check out. I've been on the Internet all day booking airline, hotel, and restaurant reservations. What did you do this afternoon?"

I didn't tell Lena that we knew the date our child was going to come into this world. I was dying to, but held off. I couldn't handle any wrath about getting a C-section right now, especially because since making my decision to have one, all I feel is relief. It *feels* like the right decision.

"I spent my afternoon shopping for maxi pads. I bought hundreds of maxi pads," I told Lena.

"What? Why did you buy so many? Why do you even need maxi pads?"

"Because supposedly I need maxi pads after giving birth. It's on the list my doctor gave me of things I have to bring to the hospital. I haven't bought maxi pads in fifteen years. I have no idea what brand or type of maxi pads is good, so I bought eight different varieties. Long ones, short ones, thick ones, thin ones, daytime ones, night-time ones, light flow ones . . ."

"Okay, okay. I get it. You know what type of maxi pad you should get?"

Crap. Does the unsolicited advice apply even to maxi pads? Will it never end?

"What kind should I get?"

"The black ones. You know the ones that everyone was writing about a year ago? The fashionable black maxi pad?"

"Lena, I don't care what color the maxi pad is, or what kind of maxi pads are in style. If you're wearing a maxi pad, you cannot feel sexy. I also have to buy new underwear. All my underwear are thongs."

"Point taken. Can we talk about what clothes I should pack for New York, and how many pairs of shoes would be too many pairs of shoes to bring?"

"Why? Are you bored of maxi pad talk already? Say it ain't so."

SEPTEMBER 24

Knowing the birthdate of your child is like having a deadline: you know exactly when you have to be prepared for it. I'm inherently a procrastinator, which means I leave everything to the last minute. I can't function, either, *unless* I leave everything until the last minute. If my editor assigns me a story due the following Monday, you can bet I'll be staying up all Sunday night to finish it.

But a baby, I think, is different from a newspaper article. A baby can't understand "Sorry I'm running a bit late. You'll get it no later than noon. I promise!" like my editor does. A baby can't really wait for diapers—this much I know. A baby can't wait to be fed—this much I also know. A baby can't be naked forever—this I know, too. And the hospital won't let you leave until you have a car seat for the baby. I've made a list of things we need to buy before the baby comes home, with the help of Ronnie, who had five minutes of quiet time after she plopped her brats—I mean kids—in front of the television.

HARDWARE
1. Car seat
2. Bottles and sterilizer for bottles
3. Bathtub
4. Nail clippers
5. Stroller
6. Thermometer
7. Baby hairbrush
8. Diaper Genie

SOFTWARE

1. Baby towels
2. Blankets
3. Sleepers
4. Undershirts
5. Hats
6. Lotions, soaps, oils
7. Diapers
8. Formula
9. Wet wipes

STUFF FOR MY HOSPITAL STAY

1. Socks
2. Underwear
3. Sweatclothes/pajamas
4. Presents for nurses and doctors
5. More maxi pads?

THINGS TO DO

1. Clean baby room/clean closets to make space for baby stuff
2. Unpack the suitcases I brought with me moving here
3. Buy an iPod (because I want one)

SEPTEMBER 25

7:00 p.m.

The fiancé and I can't have a conversation anymore without the words "baby" or "pregnancy." I worry that I'm boring him with the constant baby/pregnancy talk. I'm not going to talk about being pregnant or about the baby for the next three weeks. I'm going to be my old, charming self. I *can* not talk about the baby, can't I? I have other things to talk about, don't I? We can talk about my job, or his job, or gossip about our friends, or books we have read (rather, want to read), or movies we've seen (rather, want to see). Our lives do not revolve solely around me being pregnant and us becoming parents.

7:12 p.m.

Our lives revolve solely around me being pregnant and us becoming parents.

"I can't wait for this to be over," I tell the fiancé. Damn. I wasn't supposed to talk about being pregnant for three weeks! I lasted almost fifteen minutes.

"Why?" answers the fiancé. "So you can be hot again?"

What? What? What?

"I knew it! I knew it! I knew you no longer thought I was hot! By asking if I can't wait to be hot again, what you're really saying is that I'm not hot right now!"

"You know what I mean. I didn't mean it like that."

"Yes, you used to think I was hot and now you don't. I know exactly how you meant it," I say, starting to bawl.

Wait . . . Why isn't the fiancé trying to comfort me? I'm crying! Why is he just staring at me?

Shouldn't he be working his way over to me and giving me a hug?

"Aren't you g-g-going to t-t-try and ch-ch-cheer m-m-me up?" I sob. "I'm c-c-crying here!"

"I think you might just need a good cry."

Clearly the fiancé can't wait for this to be over as much as I can't wait for this to be over. I suppose I have cried a lot—is almost every day a lot?—throughout these past few months. He's not even attempting to cheer me up anymore.

"F-f-fine. I'm g-g-going to take a sh-sh-shower."

"That's a good idea. That will make you feel better, I'm sure."

8:00 p.m.

"AHHHHHH!!!!!"

"What now? What now?" the fiancé cries out, racing into the washroom, where I have just got out of the shower.

"This towel doesn't wrap around me anymore! Does it wrap around you, or did your cleaning lady shrink it by accident?"

"Um, it still wraps around me," the fiancé says, hesitantly.

"AHHHHHH!!!!"

"Don't worry. I have some extra-large ones in the closet. Give me a sec and I'll bring one to you. Please don't cry anymore."

The fucking towel doesn't fit around me anymore. I am *that* big. AHHHHHH!!!!

It hit me today that the woman I once was is now gone. I remember a time when I would not even blow-dry my hair in front of the fiancé, let alone be seen putting on deodorant while he was in the same room. I remember a time when I used to think those things were too personal to do in front of a man. There was a time too when I'm sure the fiancé didn't know I ever got my period, didn't know that I was capable of having gas or of eating as much as a family of six eats for dinner or of looking like I've given up on life. And now I've made the fiancé take me to a department store so I can buy some underwear to go with my new supply of maxi pads.

"Please tell me you're going to throw those out after you get out of the hospital," the fiancé says, taking in my armful of big, ugly cotton underwear. I chose the cheapest underwear in three different sizes—how am I to know what will fit my body after the baby comes out?—knowing they will be tossed out as soon as humanly possible.

"Don't worry. In my mind, they are already in the garbage. Do you think we can stop in at the drugstore on the way home?"

"Why? What do you need?"

"Some maxi pads." Welcome to the world where I'm now also comfortable talking about feminine hygiene products with the fiancé.

"Haven't you bought like twelve packs already?"

God, can a woman not buy maxi pads without being questioned?

"Yes, but then Ronnie told me about this other kind. She says that this brand is the only way to go," I tell him.

"Okay, but this is your last trip to buy maxi pads. And don't even think about asking me to take you underwear shopping again. You now own more ugly underwear than most women do in a lifetime."

It gets worse. I'm even discussing things with the fiancé that I wouldn't be comfortable talking about with my closest girlfriends.

"I have to tell you something," I tell him, when we get home. "I need to tell someone and I would tell Ronnie but I haven't been able to get in touch with her. It's really bothering me."

"What? Is something wrong?"

"No, it's just that something weird is happening to my, um, my vagina."

"What?"

"Well, it's all puffy. I have a puffy vagina."

"Is that normal?"

"I think so. I think it's because all the blood is going down there or something."

"It's your body getting ready to give birth."

"Yeah, I guess so." The fiancé starts laughing.

"And, um, I can barely wipe myself anymore after going to the washroom. I can't bend over with my big belly!"

"You are too funny," the fiancé says, still laughing.

I'm glad he thinks so. I'm just hoping the old me comes back when this is all over. I wouldn't even want to date the woman I've become, let alone marry her.

SEPTEMBER 27

3:30 a.m.

The fiancé will not wake up.

"Hey, I just had a nightmare," I say, speaking into his face.

"What? Hmmm."

"Hey! I just had a nightmare!"

"What was it about?" the fiancé mumbles.

"Oh, never mind. I don't really remember anyway."

I do remember. It was one of the strangest dreams I have ever had. It was like I was on an acid trip. He wouldn't believe me even if I told him. I dreamed that the baby was trying to get out of my body. But this baby had twelve legs, like an alien, and was trying to kick through my stomach. What if this means my baby is deformed? I should never have smoked so many cigarettes.

9:00 a.m.

I hate when people tell me about their dreams. When people start out a conversation with "I had the strangest dream last night," you know you're going to hear all about it. But the dream of giving birth to an alien child really freaked me out. I had to tell someone.

"Don't worry," Ronnie says, after I tell her about my nightmare. "I remember that at one of those parenting classes I took they said crazy dreams during pregnancy were really normal. And dreams about alien babies were common."

"Really. They specifically told you that having dreams about alien babies was normal?"

"Yes, I swear. It happens to a lot of women."

Well, at least I know I'm normal. I just pray my baby is.

SEPTEMBER 28

7:00 a.m.

"Pancakes! Pancakes! Get out of bed, sleepy head. Me want pancakes! Pancakes!"

"Jesus, Beck. What time is it?"

"Pancake time!"

"Dear God."

"Let's go to Phil's. Please?"

"Can I shower first?"

"No time for showers. I need pancakes now! Pancakes! Pancakes!"

"All right. All right. Is this going to happen every Sunday? How many more Sundays until you give birth?"

"Whatever. Let's go!"

The fiancé is obsessed with strollers. For a man, I realize, buying a stroller is like buying a car. Wheels are wheels are wheels. He forced me to sit in front of the computer today while he showed me eight different types of strollers on the Internet. When did strollers get so fancy? They all have cup holders. Some have cellphone holders. The fiancé was talking about the traction some stroller wheels have. "I've been researching strollers for weeks," he tells me. He has? Where did he find the time? "There are the Peg Peregos, which a ton of people use. But they are heavy and cumbersome. There are also the Maclaren ones, which look good and are a little lighter. But I think you'll really love the Bugaboo Frog. It's the one Ethan Hawke uses," he continues.

"Ooooh. That's cool," I tell him, perking up.

"Yeah, I'd thought you'd like that. I'm going to do some more research." The fiancé, it seems, is spending more time researching strollers than he did researching his car. At least he's into strollers. Can being into fatherhood be far behind? Maybe he's actually getting excited about all this?

SEPTEMBER 30

Busy day today. It began with a visit to Dr. Bono's office for my checkup.

"I'm a tad worried about getting a C-section now. I've been watching *A Baby Story* and *Maternity Ward* and I've seen several C-sections and each one looked bloody and violent," I told him. I've been spending my afternoons lying in bed, which is what happens when you have gained almost half your original weight and don't want to leave your bed, except for the twice-an-hour visits to the kitchen for Rice Krispie squares.

"Well, that's a mistake," Dr. Bono huffed.

"What?"

"You do realize they play up those operations for television."

"They do?"

"Of course they do. You'll be fine. It is a major operation, but you will be fine. Stop watching those shows."

"Okay."

I think Dr. Bono is starting to get me.

I also met the nanny for the first time. She is excited to work for us. She is thirty-five and very pretty.

"Make sure your nanny isn't too good-looking," Ronnie had warned.

"Why?"

"I've heard too many horror stories about husbands hooking up with their nannies."

"Come on. Really?"

"Really. I heard of one man who actually got the nanny pregnant."

"You've got to be joking!"

"I'm not. And make sure she doesn't steal from you. I have so many friends who have gone through so many nannies. Some weren't nice enough to their children, some stole clothes right from their closets, and one of my friends noticed that the change in her change drawer was dwindling day after day."

"Ronnie! The nanny hasn't even started yet. Maybe I should wait until she does before accusing her of being a thief," I told her.

"Just pay attention."

I'm worried that I won't be able to deal with having a stranger with me in the fiancé's condo all day long. He gets to get out and go to the office. I don't have an office to go to. I will technically be taking maternity leave, for at least four months, but have worked out an arrangement with my bosses. I can still write for the paper whenever I want, and I will get a paid day off for each story upon my return. But I've always worked out of the house. What if the nanny disturbs me while I'm working? Am I allowed to hang out with the nanny and the baby whenever I want to? How do I boss around a nanny? I have only ever *had* bosses. I've never *been* one. I don't know how to boss around people who are older than me—except the fiancé, and even that doesn't always work.

"What time would you like me to start every day?" the nanny asked.

"I don't know," I answered her. "What time do you usually start?"

"Well, it's up to you. You're my employer," she responded. Okay, this is going to take some getting used to. And what if my baby ends up liking the nanny more than me? And did I mention how *skinny* the nanny is? She must be a size 0. I hate her.

OCTOBER 1

11:30 p.m.

"Beck? Are you there?"

"Yes, I'm here. Where else would I be?"

"It looks like you've built yourself a fortress. For a minute, I thought you had left the bed."

"Nope, I'm right here beside you."

"I can't see you."

"I can't see you either. But this is the only way I can get comfortable."

I am lying in bed, trying to fall asleep. I've positioned six pillows under my head and along my sides, and between my legs. No matter how many pillows I have around me, no matter what position I put them in, I cannot get comfortable. I can no longer lie flat on my back. I can't breathe when I lie flat on my back.

"Do you need that?" I ask the fiancé.

"What?"

"That pillow under your head."

"How many pillows do you already have there?"

"Six."

"Well, yes, I need this *one* pillow," the fiancé tells me.

"We need more pillows. We're going to have to buy more pillows," I grumble.

"But you have *six* pillows. How many do you need?"

"I don't know. I can't get comfortable. My lower back is killing me. My upper back is killing me. My legs are killing me. My ribs are killing me. My breasts are killing me. Every part of my body is killing me. I'm not going to last! I'm not going to last!"

"You're doing great. You have less than a month to go. Really, I'm so proud of you. I love you."

"Do you love me enough to give me your pillow?"

"I need this pillow. Do you want me to bring you one from the couch?"

"Okay. Thanks. That would be great. And on your way back, can you grab me one of those heartburn pills?"

OCTOBER 2

I tried talking to Ronnie today. It's been a while.

"Ronnie! It's me," I said into the phone. It's rare for Ronnie to pick up immediately. It felt nice to hear her voice. That was until I *really* heard her voice.

"Hey! How are you, Mama! Wait one minute?" she asked.

In the background, her children were screaming as if they had just been in a haunted house.

"I'M GOING TO COUNT TO THREE!" Ronnie yelled out. "AND IF YOU AREN'T QUIET THEN YOU'RE ALL GOING TO YOUR ROOMS. ONE! TWO! THREE! Okay, I'm back. So how are you—Oh, can you hold on a second? I TOLD YOU NOT TO TOUCH THAT! Okay, I'm back. So what's—Oh God, hold on one more time. IF YOU KIDS CAN'T BEHAVE THEN YOU'RE NOT GOING TO BE ALLOWED IN THE TOY ROOM. I'M ON THE PHONE LONG DISTANCE! Okay, can you believe how loud it is in here? I swear I'm going to lose it. OKAY! THAT'S IT. I'M COMING DOWN THERE RIGHT NOW!"

"Ronnie, why don't you call me later?"

"Aren't you excited about becoming a mother? This is what happens to babies when they turn into children. You have this to look forward to. I'M GOING TO BE THERE IN THREE SECONDS!"

God, I have such a headache.

OCTOBER 4

"What are those on your feet?" the fiancé asks.

"Slippers."

"They're, uh, they're, uh, *very* nice."

"Can I get away with going out in public in these?" The fiancé and I are headed out to dinner. We don't go fancy anymore. We go casual. "We're just going for Vietnamese food, right? I don't have to look good. And my feet are really swollen. None of my shoes fit!"

"Sure. You can wear whatever."

"I'm just worried that people are going to think you broke me out of a mental hospital. It's not every day you see a woman out to dinner wearing red velvet slippers. I have to put *something* on my feet."

"Beck, you're pregnant. You can wear anything you want. No one will care. And you look kind of cute in slippers."

"No, I look like I escaped from a mental institution," I say, tearing up.

"No one will care. They'll understand."

It's true. When you're this pregnant, you can get away with wearing anything. And it's appropriate that I'm wearing slippers. Pregnancy does make you crazy. I feel like I'm going crazy.

OCTOBER 5

7:00 a.m.

"Pancakes! Pancakes! Get out of bed, sleepy head. Me want pancakes! Pancakes!"

"Jesus, Beck. What time is it?"

"Pancake time!"

"Dear God. Not again. Seriously, how many more Sundays before you have the baby?"

Didn't cry today. Maybe my pregnant hormones have gone into remission?

OCTOBER 6

Did not cry again today. I deserve a medal.

OCTOBER 7

6:30 p.m.
The fiancé is reading the paper. I'm half watching television.
"What day is it?" I ask.
"It's October 7th."
"How many more days left?"
"Eight more days."
"I'm not going to last."
"You're going to last."
"I'm not going to last."
"You will last."

6:32 p.m.
"What day is it now?" I moan.
"Beck, it's been two minutes since you asked. It's still October 7th."
"Oh. Minutes now seem like days. I'm not going to last."
"You will last," he answers, flipping the page, not looking up.

6:33 p.m.
"Is it still the same day?"
"Yes! Can I please read my paper?"

6:36 p.m.

"Is it—"

"Yes! Yes! Yes!" the fiancé huffs, picking up the paper and heading into the kitchen.

I cry. So much for my non-crying roll.

Midnight

One more week left, and I've had an epiphany. The question isn't so much why people get pregnant. I understand why women have the urge to have children. Like I've said, the biological clock ticking away is not a myth. You wake up suddenly one day and there's a need to have a baby. The question is, why would anyone want to get pregnant *again*?

This morning is my last examination before Dr. Bono performs the C-section on me next week. It's all happening so quickly, yet so slowly. It's like looking forward to a really good date. The week seems so long leading up to the date, but once it arrives it seems as though there was not enough time to prepare.

"So, um, you're not going out partying the night before my C-section next week, right?" I ask Dr. Bono while the fiancé looks at me with horror. "I mean, you're not going to go drinking at a pub or anything like that. I want you to be well rested before my operation."

"Well, obstetricians are notorious for being insomniacs," Dr. Bono answers. Not the right answer, Dr. Bono. Not the right answer.

"Oh."

"But, no, I'm not going to go drinking the night before," he says, shaking his head. "Don't worry."

Should I remind him that there are a few people who will really, really miss me if I die on his operating table? I'd better not.

I now weigh 139 pounds. This baby had better weigh at least 20 pounds.

"Don't worry," says the nurse on our way out. "He does beautiful stitching. You'll barely notice the scar."

Phew. At least that's one thing I don't have to worry about. I still want to get into bikinis one day. If that will ever be possible.

OCTOBER 9

Though I wanted to continue working right up until I give birth—I had planned to start my maternity leave the day I give birth—I realize that this is impossible.

"You know those stories I promised to do?" I tell my editor, a woman who has no children. "Well, you're not going to get any of them. I can't do anything anymore. I'm too uncomfortable to sit in front of my computer for more than five minutes, and my brain is mush." I have unfinished stories on a matchmaking school and on a hip designer in town, and another feature on trendy nail polishes, none of which are going to get done. I'm past the point of feeling bad about letting my editors down. I'm really too tired to concentrate on anything.

"Well, I understand that you get your brain back two years after giving birth," she tells me.

"Great."

I decide to call my colleague Sheila to get caught up on office gossip. I'm not too tired to do that.

"Hi. I'm sorry, I'm not in the office until October 22nd. I'm away in Switzerland on assignment," says her voice mail. "I'll get back to you upon my return."

Switzerland! What's Sheila doing in Switzerland for work? Damn. That could have been me.

Talking on the phone doesn't require any brain power at all. I call Sara today to tell her how my career is going down the tube. Maybe she's worried too, seeing as she's also going on maternity leave in a couple of months. Misery loves company. Rather, pregnancy loves misery, which means pregnancy loves company.

"My ankles are huge. They are like tree trunks," she tells me. "They are so big that my husband has started calling them 'chankles'—you know, ankles that are as big as my calves. Then at night they blow up even bigger and he calls them 'thankles' because my ankles get as big as my thighs."

"That sounds awful. I feel for you. I really do."

"And my baby is breech," she continues. "Which means I'll be having a C-section."

"Hey! Just like me! Don't worry, I'll be able to tell you exactly what happens!"

"Yeah, that's true. Do you feel a little bit badly that you're not going the vaginal route?"

"No, I really don't. Why? Do you?"

"A bit. I'm not sure why. I mean, I really just want the baby to be healthy. I guess it doesn't really matter how it gets into the world."

"Exactly. I'm more worried that my career is going down the tube."

"Sexy Young Intern bugging you again?" Sara asks. She's listened to me bitch about Sexy Young Intern before.

"She's everywhere! They love her at the paper. They love her!"

"You're going to have a baby! I think once the baby is in the world, you won't care about Sexy Young Intern. You just won't."

"I hope so. I really do."

"Beck, I've got to go. I have to go find another chair to rest my chankles on."

OCTOBER 10

2:30 a.m.

"Wake up! Wake up!"

"What? What?" the fiancé asks, startled.

"We have to get the nurses and doctors presents. I totally forgot to do that. What are we going to get them? This is a nightmare! I have no time. I still have to get a pedicure and a bikini wax! There's too much to do!"

"Calm down."

"No, you don't understand. We have to get them something good. Ronnie said that was the number one thing we had to do, next to me getting a pedicure, so that the staff will be sure to treat me super nice during my hospital stay. We need to bribe them with something!"

"I said, calm down. I already ordered fifteen really nice bottles of wine for the nurses and a bottle of champagne for Dr. Bono."

"You did?"

"Yes, I did."

"Okay. And you have to make sure you give it to him BEFORE he operates on me to make sure he does a really good job. Do you promise to do that?"

"Promise," the fiancé mumbles.

"Promise again."

"Promise."

"Promise one more time."

"I promise."

"Okay, you promised three times."

"I know. I'm just not sure he'll appreciate a bottle of champagne at nine in the morning. And, Beck, you do realize you're going to a *hospital* and not the Four Seasons, right? I'm not sure how good the service will be."

"I know that. What do you think, I'm crazy or something?"

OCTOBER 11

2:30 p.m.

I can't help but hate Saturdays now. As we inch closer and closer to the birth of our baby, Saturday has become Chore Day at the mall. I hate chores. I hate malls. I can't believe I have to spend my last Saturday as a non-parent doing chores in a mall. We should be reading the *New York Times* over eggs. We should be sleeping in. We should be going to the movies. We should be doing anything but this on our last Saturday as non-parents.

"This is the second weekend in a row we've spent buying baby crap," I moan to the fiancé as we try to find a parking space. "I hate this."

"Well, we have to do it. We're running out of time."

"I know. It's just so boring. Will it never end?"

"No, it will never end. Don't you remember last weekend at the mall?" I don't want to remember last weekend's excursion.

Buying baby crap is easier when you can get everything in one place, which is why we go to the mall. The mall also has a maternity store. The Juicy Couture trackpants I have been wearing for weeks are stretched completely out of shape, they have been worn and washed so many times. "You mean you're giving birth in just over a week and you haven't had to buy any maternity clothes?" the saleslady asked me last weekend. "Yes," I told her, "but I've been dressing like this," I said, looking down with disgust at the stretched-out trackpants and one of the fiancé's XXL sweatshirts. I didn't end up buying anything, though. Nothing fit right. Nothing at all. I left a heap of maternity pants on the changing room floor and walked out before I lost it and started bawling like a baby.

Then the fiancé almost lost it at Baby Gap. We had already bought a baby bathtub, a stroller, and a car seat. We needed some baby clothes and had already bought some at Baby Roots and Baby Old Navy. We were headed back to the parking lot when we walked past Baby Gap. We couldn't not go in. But it was a mistake. By this point, we both already had Mall Brain—that feeling you get after spending way too long in recycled air. Symptoms of Mall Brain include getting hot, flushed, and edgy, and anxious for either a long nap or a tall alcoholic beverage. We had all the symptoms.

Baby Gap was packed. We had been in the store for less than a minute when the fiancé looked at me and stated in a hard voice, "I don't think I can do this today. Can we go? *Now?*" I have never been with someone on the verge of a nervous breakdown, but the fiancé looked as though he was going in that direction. He was pale, and his mouth was in a thin line.

"Yes, let's get out of here." Mall Brain was also giving me a headache.

As we walked quickly—at least, as quickly as I could walk, being a woman giving birth in four days—I took in the scene.

"Have you noticed how many strollers there are in this mall? And how many kids shopping with their parents?"

"Yes. Welcome to our future," the fiancé answered. "We are going to spend the rest of our weekends in malls."

"Don't say that," I told him. "I know it's true, but don't say that." I hadn't thought about our baby growing up until then.

"It's true," the fiancé continued. "Kids keep growing and growing, and every time our kid grows, we'll be back at the mall buying new clothes."

"Now you're trying to depress me," I told him.

But here we are again, the following Saturday, back for more punishment.

3:15 p.m.

The fiancé and I stop for a milkshake after our visit to the mall. He needs comfort food to cheer him up. I am craving something fattening.

"I was thinking that we should get a bassinet," I tell him, sucking on my chocolate shake, "so the baby can sleep anywhere for the first few weeks. You know, if we're in the living room, the baby can sleep there too."

"I was just thinking that the other day too."

"Fuck. Does that mean we have to go back to the mall?"

"Yep."

"Fuck!"

"I know. Fuck."

"And we also forgot to get detergent for the baby. Babies' clothes need special baby detergent."

"Fuck. See? I told you. We will be spending the rest of our lives in malls buying stuff for our child."

"I know. Fuck. Fuck. Fuck."

OCTOBER 12

7:00 a.m.

"Pancakes! Panc—"

"I know. I know. We have to get you pancakes. This is the last Sunday before this baby comes out of you, thank God. I am never taking you for pancakes again!"

Oh. My. God. This is our last Sunday without a baby.

I want this thing out of me. Now.

"You know," I tell the fiancé as we're at a table at Phil's, "it's customary for the father to buy the mother of his child a gift when she gives birth. Ronnie got a new car when she had her first baby."

"Oh really?" the fiancé responds. "Ronnie has a really nice husband."

"I know. Did you get me a gift?"

"Beck, it's not becoming to ask for presents."

Oh well. At least I planted the seed. If he didn't already know about the custom, at least he does now.

OCTOBER 13

This is our last Monday without a baby.

The fiancé and I bought some parenting books earlier this evening. I'm just not sure we'll have time to actually read them before the child arrives. I mean, she's coming in two days.

When we got back home, I made the mistake of checking my work e-mail. Although I've pretty much given up on working, that doesn't mean I can stop myself from checking my e-mail. How long before I get back on my feet and can work again? I'm already getting the urge to write a story. I'm already feeling out of the loop. Occasionally the boss will send out memos about recent staff changes or new hires at the paper. I received one of those. New associate sports editor, new human resources manager, and there—there, at the bottom of the list, was Sexy Young Intern. She has been hired on at the paper full-time. She's in. I'm out. My career is over.

10:00 a.m.

This is our last Tuesday ever without a baby. Tomorrow I'm going in for a C-section. Tomorrow, at this time, I will have a baby. Tomorrow, at this time, I will be a mother. Tomorrow everything changes. Right now, we have to go pick up my mother at the airport. My mother had to come in for the birth of her first grandchild. Plus a gal needs her mother around in times like these.

11:00 a.m.

I see my mother. She is heading toward the baggage claim and—gaa!—She is not—Please tell me that's not—

"Mom! Over here!"

"Well, look at you. You are definitely ready to have a baby, I see."

"Please tell me that's not the—the video camera!" I moan, not hiding the disgust in my voice. For ten years—yes, that's how old the video camera must be—I've been plotting to steal that thing and throw it out the window.

"Of course that's the video camera," she answers. "We need a video of you before giving birth, and of the baby!"

And I thought being pregnant was bad. Now it's going to be on film. *Forever.* Maybe it was a mistake to ask my mother to come help out.

2:00 p.m.

After we took my mother out for lunch, she came back to our place and handed us a bag. In it was a sweater she had knitted. "It's for the baby's going-home outfit." Gaa! Two days ago, the fiancé's mother handed us a bag with the baby's going-home outfit in it. I had never even heard of a going-home outfit. I can't handle this stress right now—the day before my C-section. Someone's feelings are going to be hurt.

4:00 p.m.

Maybe I've been too hard on many of my friends during these last few months. Maybe they really do care about me. They have all called wishing me luck tomorrow. Of course, I told them all about my scheduled C-section. What did you think? That I could possibly have kept something so juicy a secret?

8:00 p.m.

The fiancé and I are back home, after having dinner with my mother and his parents, to enjoy our last *hours* as non-parents. How do you spend your last hours as a non-parent?

"Can you believe that tomorrow we're going to have a baby?" I ask him.

"No, can you?"

"No."

"It's very weird."

"It is."

"I'm still not convinced about the first name Rowan," I continue. The fiancé and I, after hours and hours of discussion, have come up with the name Rowan, stolen from an issue of *Us Weekly*. Thank you, Brooke Shields, for having a daughter named Rowan! In all our discussions over the past few weeks, Rowan was the only name we both liked (Apple never did take).

"I like it and everything, but I keep thinking that our child's name should have some real meaning," I say. "Something between you and me, like your friends who named their child after that bottle of wine they really love, Salai. That's romantic. We don't have a name with real meaning for us. I can't think of anything, either, and it's all I've been thinking about for months. We could name her after an airline, because of our long-distance relationship."

"You know we're having the baby tomorrow, right?"

"Yeah, I was thinking that . . . Well, you know how I realized I was in love with you when we were in Las Vegas at the Palm restaurant?"

"Yes."

"Well, how about the name Palmer?"

"That's not bad. Hmmm. Palmer. I like it."

"Do you like it enough to change her name to Palmer?"

"Do you?"

"I don't know. And about the middle name . . ."

"Listen, I told you the middle name is all yours. If you want the middle name to be Apple, you can have it."

"Actually, I was thinking about the name Joely, after your cousin who passed away. How do you feel about Joely?"

"I really love that."

"Okay, let's sleep on it. How should we spend our last night together without a baby?"

"Don't you have to pack for the hospital?"

Oh. Right. What a boring way to spend my last night as a non-mother.

"Yeah. I guess I better do that."

11:00 p.m.

The checklist! I can't find the checklist that Dr. Bono handed me during one of our appointments! I have no idea what to pack! The checklist had everything on it that the baby and I need for our hospital stay!

11:38 p.m.

Found the checklist crumpled in a ball in one of my jacket pockets. Phew. I lay out one suitcase for me, and one suitcase for our baby. I'm a notorious overpacker. When we went to Hawaii for ten days, I packed enough clothes for a month, or maybe two. But you never know. It could have snowed. Better to be prepared than not prepared. I am going to be in the hospital for three days. I pack sixteen pairs of underwear, five pairs of sweats, five long-sleeved shirts, five T-shirts, eight pairs of socks, a new bottle of shampoo, a new bottle of conditioner (there had better be a shower in my room!), a new bar of soap and new deodorant, four packs of maxi pads, and two pillows. For the baby, I pack nine sleepers, five undershirts, four blankets, six hats, and a pack of diapers.

"You do know you're only going to be there for three days?" the fiancé asks, coming into the bedroom, where I'm on the floor, rolling everything into small balls so it will all fit into the suitcases.

"I know. But the list was kind of stingy."

"How many diapers do you have there?"

"Eighty."

"Eighty? *Eighty?*"

"Well, do you know how many times a day a baby needs to be changed?"

"No. Should we get the book out?"

"I don't even know where those books are."

"Me neither. So you're all packed then?"

"Yep."

"So we're ready then?"

"Well, I'm not sure how ready we are to have a baby, but we're definitely ready to go to the hospital. Hey, can you help me up?" I ask, sticking out my hands for a lift, hopefully for the last time.

THINGS I HAVE DONE WRONG
DURING THIS PREGNANCY

1. Ate like shit for nine months.
2. Had four Benedryls to help me sleep. They didn't work.
3. Smoked the occasional cigarette.
4. Have yet to talk to my stomach, aside from telling the baby to stop moving while I'm trying to sleep. Have not played any soothing music to my stomach either, aside from putting airplane headsets on it for one minute, just to see if they would fit.
5. Did not lie with my legs up for ten minutes a day to keep varicose veins away.
6. Drank at least a couple dozen Diet Cokes. Had one large, caffeinated coffee a day.
7. Watched way too many hours of reality television.
8. Have not worked out in months. Have barely even left the house in the last month.
9. Constantly bitched and moaned.
10. Stressed out every day over work, Cute Single Man, my future.
11. Always woke up somehow sleeping on my stomach. Perhaps dented the baby's head?

THINGS I DID RIGHT
DURING THIS PREGNANCY

1.   Ate three salads.
2.   Drank no alcohol (except half a glass of wine on my birthday).
3.   Still haven't bounced on a trampoline.
4.   Watched way too many hours of reality television. (Perhaps the baby can be the next American Idol or winner of *Survivor*?)

WEDNESDAY, OCTOBER 15

6:00 a.m.

The fiancé just got out of the shower. He has to head to his office this morning to close a deal or do whatever it is he does at work. He'll be coming to pick me up at 8 a.m. His deal had better close on time.

One of my colleagues once told me how he brought his laptop into the hospital room while his wife was in labor. He set up his computer on the tray table over her bed, plugged it into the socket on the wall, and proceeded to write his column. I asked him if his wife got mad because he continued to work while she was in labor. "Well, it was taking a while," he answered. Still, because of this colleague I had to make sure the fiancé would not be working while I was getting my C-section.

"You're not bringing your BlackBerry into the

delivery room, right?" I asked him yesterday. "Because I will get very pissed off if you start answering your e-mail while I'm in surgery."

"Of course I'm not going to be checking e-mail while you're in surgery."

"And you're not going to bring your cellphone in either, right?"

"Of course not," the fiancé answered, laughing.

"Not even on vibrate, right?"

"Right."

"Because that buzzing really annoys the hell out of me."

7:00 a.m.

I just showered and blow-dried my hair.

7:30 a.m.

I am not allowed to eat breakfast. I haven't eaten anything since midnight last night. I'm starving.

I light up a cigarette from a secret stash I have hidden in a kitchen cupboard. I inhale. What damage can it do now? Plus, I'm nervous.

8:00 a.m.

Where is the fiancé? I'm all ready to go. Where is he? Has he forgotten about me? Has he forgotten we're having a *baby* today?

8:15 a.m.

We're lost. The fiancé has decided to take a new, "faster" route to avoid rush-hour traffic. Why is it that new, "faster" routes always get you lost? I knew we were headed for trouble when I said, "Hey, is this the way we get to the hospital?" and the fiancé answered, "I think this route will also get us there."

"You think? *You think?*"

"Don't worry. We'll get there. Don't freak."

Don't freak. Trying not to freak.

"I think it will be very wrong to be late for a C-section. This isn't like being late for a restaurant reservation."

"We won't be late."

"We have to be there in ten minutes!"

"We won't be late."

"We have to be there in nine minutes!"

8:30 a.m.

Phew. We made it.

8:46 a.m.

"Oh, I almost forgot to give you this," I say, handing the fiancé a crumpled piece of paper.

"What is it?"

"It's a list of my friends' phone numbers. You have to call them after and tell them what happens. It's not that exciting since most of them know I'm having the baby today and that it's a girl, but they might want to know the weight."

"Okay. Funny how this is the one thing that no one had to remind you to do."

8:59 a.m.

Time to have a baby. I am now naked, except for socks and a blue hospital gown (which, of course, does not do up at the back), waiting in the "prep" room. The fiancé is in scrubs, accessorized with an ugly paper hat over his hair and matching ugly paper slippers to put over his shoes.

The anesthetist comes in to introduce himself and explain how the needle goes into my spine for the epidural and that I'll be frozen from my breasts down to my toes. I'll still be able to move my arms. He is super friendly and puts me at ease immediately. He tells me his wife has had two C-sections and she was fine. He tells me he'll be at my side the entire time.

I have given my last pee sample. My blood pressure has been taken for the last time. An IV is hooked up to my wrist. I am being wheeled to the delivery room.

9:00 a.m.

The operating room—or, rather, the delivery room—is very cold. I'm shivering. There are half a dozen people in scrubs standing around. Where is Dr. Bono? The fiancé has been directed to a viewing booth where he has to watch me get the epidural. After that's done he can come in the room and hold my hand during the C-section. I see him watching me through the glass. I miss him. I need him beside me right now. He gives me the thumbs-up sign, which is all he can do to show his support from where he is watching. I hate the thumbs-up sign almost as much as I hate people who want to high-five me.

Something is going to fuck up. I'm going to end up paralyzed. I know it, even though the super-friendly anesthetist has told me that the chances of that happening are one in a million. I could be that one in a million. It *is* possible.

9:10 a.m.

Gaa! Who is this woman armed with a needle coming toward me? I shouldn't have looked at the needle. It is huge. That's going to hurt, I think. That's going to *hurt*.

"This is another anesthetist. She'll be helping me out," the super-friendly anesthetist tells me. Do not freak, Beck. Do not freak. They wouldn't let her stick that needle in me if she didn't know what she was doing, right?

If the fiancé does not stop giving me the thumbs-up sign, I'm going to hurt someone.

9:11 a.m.

OWW! The pain! "That really, really hurts," I tell the super-friendly anesthetist, who is behind me with the female anesthetist. I'm not being super friendly. I start to cry. "OWW. Seriously . . . Is it supposed to hurt like that?" I ask, sobbing. "It really, really hurts."

The female anesthetist takes the needle out from my back. "We'll try it again," she says.

The super-friendly male anesthetist starts giving directions to the female anesthetist. "Oh, you were putting it in a little high. You should try a little lower down in her back," he tells her. GAA! Wait! Is she practicing on me? Do they not know that I can *hear* them? Do they not know that this is my spine? I want to scream out to the male anesthetist, "YOU DO IT! YOU DO IT! I AM NOT A GUINEA PIG! I TRUST YOU!" But I don't want to be a prima donna. I don't want to be a brat. Instead, I really start bawling, resorting to my "tears work" theory.

"Okay, you know what?" the super-friendly male anesthetist says, seeing my distress. "I'm going to do it."

God is listening. Thank God. The needle goes into my back effortlessly.

9:30 a.m.

I'm lying on the operating bed. I can't feel my bum. My legs are tingling, getting more and more numb by the nanosecond. The fiancé comes in and grabs my hand. A sheet is drawn right at my neck level so I won't be able to see what happens on the other side. Dr. Bono comes in. At least I think it's Dr. Bono. I can't tell because this man is wearing scrubs and a face mask, which covers everything but his eyes.

"Are we ready to go?" Phew. I hear his accent. It's Dr. Bono.

"We're ready," everyone else in the room answers in unison.

It's definitely too late to turn back now. I look into the fiancé's eyes. I love you, I think. I'd better be frozen. I'd better not feel *anything*.

9:35 a.m.

"Did you just feel that?" the super-friendly anesthetist asks me.

"No. Feel what?"

"It's good you didn't feel anything. The doctor just did something really nasty to you."

What?? What was Dr. Bono doing behind the sheet? Nasty does not sound good.

9:40 a.m.

"You're going to feel some pressure very soon," Dr. Bono calls out from behind the sheet. To get the baby out, he says, he uses his elbow to push her down the opening he has cut in my lower stomach. How can a baby fit out through a six-inch opening, the length of the cut Dr. Bono said he would make? Not going to worry about it. Not going to worry about it.

9:43 a.m.

"Ow. I can feel the pressure," I cry out.

"You're doing great," the super-friendly anesthetist tells me. "Everything is going great."

"How much longer? How much longer?"

"We're almost done," says the super-friendly anesthetist.

"You're doing great," says the female anesthetist.

"You're doing great," says the fiancé. At least now people are telling me that I'm "doing great" as opposed to "looking great." I do not let go of the fiancé's hand, though my palms are super sweaty. Or are those his palms that are sweaty?

9:58 a.m.

"She's coming out now," someone says. "Here she comes." This is my last second being a non-mother.

9:59 a.m.

WAAAA!! I hear the scream of a baby. Dr. Bono holds my baby up over the sheet so I can see her. That's *my* baby? She looks slimy and wet and pink and squiggly.

She's perfect.

"Time of birth?" someone calls out.

"9:59 a.m.," answers Dr. Bono. A nurse takes my baby to a corner in the room to check her out and clean her up.

WAAAA!! That's me crying now. The fiancé kisses me. I kiss him back. I'm crying, this time because I'm happy and relieved. I feel . . . I feel . . . happier than I ever thought I could ever feel. Ever. I have never known happiness like this, and I am savoring it, like a juicy first kiss. This feeling is better than any first kiss. I am convinced I can never feel this happy again. I want to remember everything about this moment.

The fiancé keeps kissing me and kissing me. I want to inhale him, too. But where is my baby?

"Can you go check on her?" I ask him, and he goes to where they are cleaning her off. I have the overwhelming urge to make sure everything is okay. This must be the maternal instinct that everyone told me would kick in.

"Do we have a name yet?" someone calls out.

"Rowan Joely," I call out. Rowan Joely. Rowan Joely. My daughter.

10:05 a.m.

Baby Rowan is in my arms, wrapped in a blanket with a cap on her head. She fits perfectly. She is beautiful. The fiancé is looking down at us, beaming. We kiss again.

The sheet is still up. Dr. Bono is taking out the placenta and stitching me up. At least that's what I think he's supposed to be doing now. I don't even notice.

10:12 a.m.

I'm in the recovery room. A nurse has taken Baby Rowan and is weighing and measuring her. She weighs 7 pounds, 3 ounces.

The fiancé's parents come into the room with my mother. They all gather around the baby. They aren't paying any attention to me. Baby Rowan is everything. I'm still weepy. The fiancé has taken off his gown and cap. I notice that there are huge sweat stains on his shirt under his arms. He's forgotten to take off the paper shoes. Camera clicks and flashes are going off at breakneck speed. The fiancé is holding my hand.

"We have a baby," I say to him. He too looks teary.

"We have a baby," he responds, holding my hand even tighter.

Baby Rowan is again in my arms. I never want to let her go.

10:00 p.m.

A nurse comes into the room and kicks out my mother and the fiancé's parents. The fiancé is allowed to stay as long as he wants, or as long as I want him to, which is forever. The nurse tells me she's taking out my catheter—I didn't even know I had one—and helps me to the washroom. Walking to the washroom, only a couple of feet away, is difficult. I'm getting caught in the tubes and IV, which pump liquids in to keep me hydrated. And my stomach feels clenched as tight as a fist. I can finally feel my bum and my legs again. I'm not paralyzed, thank God.

The nurse helps me sit on the toilet seat. "You're going to try peeing on your own now," she says. I see I'm wearing disposable one-size-fits-all mesh panties. How did those get on me? And who put that huge maxi pad in there? The nurse takes off my underwear and changes my maxi pad for me. Ronnie is right. I don't care that a stranger is watching me pee and changing my maxi pad. My baby is healthy and lying in a crib beside my bed.

THINGS THAT NEVER HAPPENED
DURING MY PREGNANCY

1. My hair never got super shiny.
2. Strangers never touched my pregnant belly without asking.
3. My fingernails never grew.
4. I did not work out to the very end, nor did I exercise after six months.
5. I did not entirely stop smoking.
6. I did not enjoy being pregnant.

THINGS EVERY WOMAN SHOULD
KNOW ABOUT GIVING BIRTH

1. Presents do work on hospital staff. Nurses did treat me nicer after receiving bottles of wine and boxes of chocolate.
2. You can wear socks during delivery—no need for a pedicure. A bikini wax is a good idea, though.
3. You will not care once the baby is born how many humiliating positions strangers see you in.
4. It is the most rewarding thing you will ever do. Whether you have a vaginal birth or a C-section, the first time you see your baby will be the happiest moment of your life.
5. Take whatever drugs they offer you.

9:00 a.m.

Though I have done no real physical work in giving birth to Baby Rowan—no pushing, no huffing, no puffing, no punching the fiancé in the face—I am exhausted. I feel more tired than I've ever felt after finishing spin class. I feel like I've just run a marathon, and I don't do marathons. But I'm too excited to sleep or nap for more than a half hour at a time. What if I miss something? Baby Rowan *is* better than any reality TV show. I can't stop staring at her. She's so small. Look at her tiny feet! Look how much hair she has! Look how beautiful she is! Look how cute her hands are! Who the hell does she look like? Plus, have you ever tried to sleep in a maternity ward? At any given time there is at least one baby crying somewhere. Which is the problem with babies. Just because it's lights out at 10:00 p.m. in the hospital doesn't mean the babies shut up. Babies don't understand time or that their mothers have just given birth to them and are exhausted.

One of the nurses showed the fiancé and me how to change diapers yesterday. It's easy. What was I freaking out about? Only an idiot couldn't figure out how to put on Pampers. The fiancé actually seems to enjoy changing Baby Rowan's diapers. What is wrong with him?

Me? I enjoy feeding her the most. The hospital provides mini bottles of ready-made formula.

I hold the nipple up to Baby Rowan's perfect miniature mouth and she sucks away immediately. Such a smart baby! She knows exactly what to do! Could it be that I have just given birth to a future Nobel Prize winner? She falls soundly asleep for a couple of hours after every feeding. I don't turn on the television the fiancé has ordered for me in the room. I can miss an episode of *The West Wing* to watch Baby Rowan. I feel proud. This is my greatest accomplishment.

"Everything going okay in here?" says one of the friendly, motherly nurses walking into my room. (They are all friendly and motherly. It would be wrong not to be friendly and motherly if you work on a maternity ward, after all.)

"Yes. Everything is fine. Do you think I could get some more codeine pills?"

"It's been four hours. So yes. I'll bring you some in a minute," the nurse responds.

I'm not sure if I still need them. But why chance it? Plus I kind of enjoy the woozy feeling they give me. Despite Ronnie's warnings that I would not be able to hold my baby let alone walk after the C-section, I can and do. I'm not going to let a little thing like a C-section get in the way of holding my baby! I'm not even in that much pain unless I try to jump out of bed, which I can't really do anyway. The nurses have told me that I'm recovering extremely well. Maybe I'm just lucky. Of course, I play up what little pain I have— just a bit—so the fiancé will continue fetching me ice water and sandwiches from the cafeteria downstairs. I should be pampered and waited on after giving birth! The fiancé also makes me take walks around the maternity floor with him every couple of hours. I had been told that recovery is much easier if you force yourself to walk as soon as you can after getting a C-section. It's good to walk. (I'm not paralyzed from the epidural! Yay!) I also want to check out the other babies in the ward to see how Baby Rowan measures up. She is the cutest of them all. And I'm not just saying that because I'm her mother. (Of course, I did hear another new mother holding her newborn whisper to her husband, "Jake is cuter than any baby here!" She's just plain wrong.) I also found a scale on the floor while taking a walk, which I hopped on, much to the fiancé's dismay.

"I can't believe you can't even wait to go home to weigh yourself."

I can't bear to say aloud what I weigh. Oh, the pain. Finding out what I weighed even after Baby Rowan was out of me was more painful than any C-section.

OCTOBER 18

9:00 a.m.

I'm being kicked out of the hospital. The fiancé has not come to pick me up yet. He left late last night. It can't be time to go home already! I've only known Baby Rowan for three days! I don't know what to do with a baby. What if something goes wrong? What if I drop her? What if I can't figure out how to make formula on my own or she doesn't like the formula I make her? (There are plenty of adults who hate my cooking. I even hate my cooking, which is why I don't cook! What if my baby hates the food I make her?) What if I break her neck putting on her undershirts or she suffocates in her blankets? How can they expect someone who doesn't know anything about a baby to go off on her own and take care of a baby? No, I can't leave. They can't force me to leave. (Actually they can, and they are.)

No, I'm staying here forever and everyone is just going to have to deal with it. Who am I kidding? I have to leave. I do want to take a long, hot shower in the privacy of my own home. I think I'm starting to smell. I do want to sleep in my own bed. I do want to walk around my own condo in bare feet without the fear that I'm going to catch some nasty foot disease. (The hospital is nice, but it's no Four Seasons.) Oh God. How can this be happening?

The nurses check me over one last time. "How's flow?" one of them asks me. Flow? Flow? Who's Flow? Do I know a Flow? Is this nurse mixing me up with another patient who has a friend named Flow?

"Flow? Oh, do you mean the blood coming out of me?" I couldn't believe there was blood coming out of me from Down There. No one warned me about this. I thought if you have a C-section then nothing happens Down There. But it turns out that any way you give birth, the uterus still starts shrinking back to its normal size, which makes you bleed for up to six weeks! How can a person function with so much blood loss? There's just so much blood. To say I'm disappointed in my uterus would be an understatement.

"Yes, that's what I mean."

"Fine. I mean, it's coming out of me." I'm still wearing the hospital-provided disposable one-size-fits-all mesh panties. I've moved on to my own stash of maxi pads. Thank God I have hundreds and hundreds of them.

I call the fiancé, who is still in bed. "You'd better come get me now. They're kicking me out. And I can't leave with the baby until they see the car seat."

The fiancé arrives within fifteen minutes. Together we change Baby Rowan's diaper.

We're handed pamphlets on postpartum depression, with emergency phone numbers in case I feel suicidal or can't stop crying once I get home.

"I'd better not get that," I tell the fiancé as we're packing me up. It's a bitch. I packed way too much.

"I know. I know."

"But if the last nine months are any indication, I probably will. I'm a crier."

"I know. I know. I was there, remember, when you had prepartum depression for, oh, I don't know, nine months?"

"Ha ha. Right now, though, I feel amazing about life."

"I'll keep the pamphlets handy, though. Just in case," the fiancé says.

"Let's dress Baby Rowan. What are we going to put her in? We have to put her in the outfit my mother knitted for her or else her feelings will be hurt. She spent a long time knitting that, and it's pretty damn adorable."

"But we also have to put her in the pink and white striped thing *my* mother bought her or else *her* feelings will be hurt," the fiancé says.

Baby Rowan leaves the hospital wearing the pink and white striped sleeper the fiancé's parents bought under the rainbow-colored sweater and hat set my mother knit. Baby Rowan does not match. She looks a little ridiculous, actually, as though she's dressed for a dogsled ride in the Arctic. But nothing can get me down right now. I feel like I'm on some sort of amazing high. They should bottle this feeling.

Of course, I'm still wearing men's sweatpants, which is disturbing. But, hey, I had a baby *three days ago.* Cut me some slack.

I'm a Mother. I'm Still Fat!

THINGS I DID NOT KNOW ABOUT
POST-PREGNANCY

1. I will have "flow" for up to six weeks.
2. It takes six weeks for my uterus to get back to normal size.
3. I will still look five to six months pregnant after giving birth and for who knows how long.
4. There will be a dark line from my chest down to my pubic area—totally normal, but it will take about a month to disappear.
5. You cannot eat four Big Macs a week, french fries every day, and as much junk food as your heart desires and not work out at all for nine months and still expect to fit back into your size 6 jeans again. Ever, maybe.

6. Everyone will ask for pictures. (Note to self: Learn how to e-mail photos from digital camera immediately.)
7. The cravings and the heartburn do go away, almost instantly.
8. You cannot have sex for *six weeks* after a C-section.
9. You cannot work out for *six weeks* after a C-section.

OCTOBER 20

The nanny arrives at eight o'clock this morning for her first day at work. The fiancé has decided to take the week off work. My mother is still in town. I feel as though the fiancé and I haven't had any alone time in weeks and weeks, though in reality it has been only days. Our families are always around.

So far Baby Rowan is an angel. She passes out for hours after we feed her. We have decided not to breastfeed, which, so far, is working out brilliantly. I do not feel guilty about this at all. I turned out okay and I wasn't breastfed, and so did the fiancé, who wasn't breastfed either.

The doorman at the fiancé's condo has been buzzing us nonstop. We have received dozens of gifts, gift baskets, and bouquets of flowers. I feel like I've just won an Academy Award. People do care. They do! Heather, Lena, Vivian, Shannon, Marci, Sara, and Dana all called, too, and listened

to me talk about Baby Rowan and the C-section
for as long as I wanted.

"Should I get the number? Should I get the number?"

I'm crying. Shit. The fiancé thinks I'm having a
postpartum meltdown. Maybe I am?

"Seriously. Do you think this is the postpartum
depression thing?" he continues, concerned.

I have called the fiancé on his cellphone from the
washroom in his condo, where I have gone to cry
and be alone. He was with the baby and my mother
and his parents and the nanny in the living room.

"C-c-can you c-c-come s-see me?" I cried to
the fiancé from my cellphone.

"Where are you?"

"In the w-w-washroom in the bedroom."

"What's wrong? What's wrong?"

"It's just that everyone is always around," I sob
when he comes in. "And everyone is holding my
baby more than me. And she's *my* baby!"

Ever since we arrived home, the fiancé's parents, my mother, and the nanny have been here
constantly, picking up my baby. I feel as though
I've barely touched her.

"They're super excited too, Beck. And, trust
me, next week your mother will be gone and then
my parents won't be hanging around so much, and
you'll be wishing they were here to help."

"You think?"

"Yes. They just really love her and want to hold her. But she is your baby. You can pick her up whenever you want."

"Okay. I'm going to, then. I'm going to pick her up right now."

"So you're okay now?"

"Yes."

"So you don't have postpartum depression?"

"I don't think so. At least not yet."

OCTOBER 22

Still wearing men's sweatpants. I still look six months pregnant. When is this belly going to go away?

"Beck, it's going to take longer than a week. It's going to take months."

"NO! It has to be gone by December 31st."

"What? Why? Why December 31st?"

"Um, I have a bet going with Heather. I bet her $500 that I could lose the weight by December 31st."

"You are crazy," the fiancé says. "You had nine months of pure gluttony. You ate everything and anything you wanted. It's going to take a while."

"I know. I know. You don't have to remind me. My big ass is reminder enough."

3:00 p.m.

I have not had one carbohydrate all week. I am eating only protein, fruits, and vegetables. Surprisingly, I do not miss Big Macs or french fries. I think I overdosed on McDonald's. I will never eat there again.

"Oh, you'll eat there again," Ronnie told me when I told her how good I've been with my post-pregnancy diet.

"No I won't. I'm done with McDonald's."

"When your baby can eat solid food, you'll be there at least once a week. Trust me."

I don't see it happening. It was a good relationship while it lasted, but I had to ditch Ronald eventually. He's not really my type of guy.

8:00 p.m.

My mother has left. So, too, has the video camera. Thank God. The fiancé and I are alone. Finally. It feels great, but still weird knowing there's a third human at home with us. I can't stop staring at Baby Rowan. This is the most rewarding thing I have ever done.

Gaa! Did that really come out of *my* mouth? Were all those people who kept telling me that this will be the most rewarding thing I have ever done actually right? Baby Rowan is my yummy angel.

Midnight

Baby Rowan is wailing. Do not freak. Check diaper. Hold her. Feed her. She goes back to sleep.

2:00 a.m.

Baby Rowan is screaming. Do not freak. Somehow get myself out of bed. Hold her. Change her. Feed her. Phew.

3:56 a.m.

Baby Rowan is wailing. Gaaa!! Am so tired, cannot get out of bed. Is the fiancé asleep, or just pretending to be asleep? How can he sleep through this? Get out of bed. Feed her. Change her. Rock her back to sleep.

5:00 a.m.

WAAA! Baby Rowan is the devil! The sound of a newborn wailing is an awful, awful sound. It's a much worse sound than the alarm clock going off after a sleepless night. Oh man, it's so much worse than that.

6:00 a.m.

Finally, Baby Rowan is asleep. Please let me sleep, Baby Rowan. Please let me sleep.

6:45 a.m.

ARGH!!!!! What's my name? Where am I? Who's screaming?

"Wake up!"

"I'm up. I've been up all night," the fiancé says. "I'm a wreck, I'm so tired."

"Your turn. I haven't been to sleep yet," I tell the fiancé. "I thought you were sleeping. Didn't you hear me get up all those times?"

"I did. Of course I did. I have to work today. I can't believe I have to work on one hour of sleep."

"I have such a bad headache," I tell the fiancé.

"Go take some Advil. That will help."

Right! I can now take Advil without fearing that my baby will have two heads. I pop three.

8:00 a.m.

The nanny arrives. Baby Rowan is sleeping like an angel. She does not wake up until noon. I spend my morning talking on the phone to friends and my mother.

"You know what you have to do?" Ronnie says. "You have to get her on a schedule. Every night do the same thing. Bathe her and feed her at the same time, so she knows it's bedtime."

"You know what you have to do?" my mother says. "Make sure she's in a dark, quiet room." Sheesh. Does my mother really think I have

365

been blasting AC/DC and putting on a light show while trying to put Baby Rowan to sleep?

"You know what I've read?" says Heather. "That babies like those swing things. Maybe you should buy her a swing."

"Maybe it's her formula," suggests Vivian.

Argh. Pregnancy does end. But apparently the unsolicited advice does not.

5:00 p.m.

Cute Single Man sent me an e-mail congratulating me on Baby Rowan after reading the paper. I had written a story about Baby Rowan coming into this world by C-section—the wave of the future, I'm convinced, especially since *Vogue* published an article about the same topic. Once it's in *Vogue,* it's like the law. And having a C-section really wasn't that bad. I would recommend it to any woman. I'm still walking quite slowly and I have to sit down and get up a little more carefully, but each day it gets easier and easier. Except when I sneeze. When I sneeze and my whole body shakes (I sneeze passionately), it hurts. But, hey, I don't sneeze all that often. I still can't carry anything heavy. (Thank God my baby is not even 8 pounds. Plus, I don't like carrying heavy items anyway. Who does?)

I wrote another feature about designer baby wear and how it is also possible to spend more on a stroller than on a used car. It is also possible to still have a career, I think, at least with a nanny around. Having a baby will be good for my career.

At least, it provides me with a ton of story ideas. (Next article? "How to Survive on Three Minutes of Sleep.") Sexy Young Intern had a piece in the paper today, too, about a new bar in town that features waitresses who dance on the bar counter, like at Coyote Ugly in New York. I didn't finish her story, which was featured prominently in the Life section. I have a baby now, and bar hopping seems, well, not so important to me anymore. She can have my old job, I think. I barely have time to read the newspaper anyway.

I send Cute Single Man an e-mail back, thanking him. I have a pang of regret. I still miss him.

OCTOBER 25

9:45 p.m.

"I'm so excited to go to bed," the fiancé tells me as he's about to brush his teeth. "I'm beat."

"Me too. I don't think I've ever been this tired," I respond. I'm already in my pajamas. "It's not even ten o'clock. I guess this is what people meant when they said a baby changes everything." I now understand why Ronnie never picks up her phone after 8:30. She is a mother, after all. I get it now.

"Yep. Isn't it rewarding?" the fiancé jokes.

"I want to have sex. I want very, very badly to have sex," I tell him. It's back. My mojo is back. Thank God. The fiancé has never looked so attractive.

"How many more weeks?"

"Three," I tell the fiancé.

Note to self: Buy condoms.

OCTOBER 26

It was a good night last night. I slept three hours straight. Sara's husband just called. She had her baby two weeks early. Her baby girl arrived last night after her water broke and he rushed her to the hospital for her C-section. He gave me the room number at the hospital.

"Congratulations!" I scream into the phone. "Baby Rowan's first girlfriend has arrived."

"Hey. Thanks so much. You're so sweet," Sara says sleepily into the phone. "She came early. Can you believe it? I didn't even have a chance to get my manicure and pedicure and haircut. I was scheduled to get it all done tomorrow."

"Oh, who cares? You have a baby girl! You're going to love it. It's going to be the most rewarding thing, you'll see. But just remember to get up and get walking ASAP. That will help you get over the C-section so much faster."

Shit. I've turned into one of the people I hate, the type that gives unsolicited advice to new parents. Well, I am a parent who has been through a C-section. Don't I know how it's done? Shouldn't I pass on my knowledge? Oh God. I've gone over to the dark side.

"You know what's weird?" I ask the fiancé while Baby Rowan is sleeping. We are wolfing down dinner (no carbs for me) for fear Baby Rowan will interrupt us before we finish.

"What?"

"Lately my parents haven't asked me about when we're going to get married. In fact, no one has asked. Has anyone asked you?"

"No. It's all about Baby Rowan now. No one cares about us anymore."

It's true. When my parents call or the fiancé's parents call, they don't ask how we are. They only ask how Baby Rowan is. It's like we don't exist.

"I still can't believe we have a child, can you?" I say to the fiancé. "It's still all so surreal."

"I know. It's like—" *WAAAA!!* Baby Rowan is awake again.

"Can you believe it now?" the fiancé yells over the wails. "I'm going to start calling her The Dictator. Because she always gets what she wants."

369

OCTOBER 28

It is time to try to start losing what has now been dubbed my Baby Rowan Behind, or the Baby Rowan Rump. I walk on a treadmill for twenty minutes. Losing this ass is going to take forever.

My breasts are slowly starting to get back to my pre-pregnancy size. That is unfortunate.

OCTOBER 29

The towel fits around my body again, I realize, stepping out of the shower. THE TOWEL FITS AROUND MY BODY AGAIN! I still have a good twenty-seven pounds to lose, however. What if it never goes away? What if I never see my old pre-pregnant body again?

"You're not planning on going back to your pre-pregnancy weight, are you?" Shannon asked me this morning when I called to say hi.

"I do plan on it. Why?"

"It's just that you were so skinny before."

Crap. Am I not allowed to have a good body and be a mother? Am I not allowed to be vain anymore?

OCTOBER 30

"I have The Fear," Lena says into the phone. She met a guy last night at a new bar in town, got drunk, and somehow they ended up kissing in the men's washroom. She doesn't remember how she got home. I laugh along with her tale. Some things never change.

Tonight I have made plans with Casey, a girl my age who is friends with the fiancé. It's time to get back out there and try to begin making a life for myself here, after bringing a new life into the world. First step, make friends.

Casey and I are going to a bar. I will have my first alcoholic drink in what seems like forever. I will not order Perrier. The nanny is sleeping over. I can't imagine waking up with a hangover and having to take care of a screaming baby. Maybe it is possible to have my old life mixed in with my new life. Who knows?

OCTOBER 31

11:00 a.m.

I've booked a ticket to come back to my hometown for a visit, with Baby Rowan. I will now be one of those people travelers moan about when they see them get on the plane with a baby. I will be a pre-boarder. Oh well. I'll be praying along with them that Baby Rowan doesn't wail the entire flight. I'm excited to see my friends and my apartment. I plan on spending at least half my new life at my apartment with Baby Rowan.

I call Heather first to make sure she keeps the first Saturday night I'm in town open for me. "My mother will babysit Baby Rowan that night," I tell her, "so we can go out and party. I don't think I can stay out super late, though."

"Right," she says. "You have to plan your nights out now. You have to worry about finding babysitters."

Right.

I call Ronnie next.

"So are you ready to have another yet?" she asks. Is she joking? Please tell me she's joking. She's got to be joking.

"No way. Never again. I love Baby Rowan to death, but I can't see myself pregnant again. Ever."

"Oh, you say that now. But you'll see. You're going to want another. Trust me on this. Wait until she smiles at you for the first time—you'll forget all about the sleepless nights and you'll want another baby."

"I don't know about that," I tell her. "But, please, next time I tell you I'm going out drinking, remind me to stop at two drinks. I'm serious. Two drinks is my limit. I don't want to have another love child."

"I don't think you'll be going out nearly as much. You're going to enjoy staying home more. You'll get tired at ten o'clock," Ronnie tells me, knowingly. "You won't ever want to drink that much again. You'll have other worries now."

Is she right? I do have other worries. My life has changed. I haven't figured out how to use the Diaper Genie yet, and the humidifier we bought for the baby room doesn't seem to work. My mother is bugging me to send pictures of the baby and she sounds jealous that the fiancé's parents get to spend so much time with the baby. I think Baby Rowan is catching her first cold, and is that baby acne on her face or a rash of some sort? When do

I start training Baby Rowan to sleep through the night, and does she have enough warm clothes? How exactly do you bathe a newborn? The fiancé is also angry with me after I asked him one too many times this morning if my ass is still fat and if my hair looks thinner. I still don't fit into any of my pre-pregnancy clothes. Maybe I should join a mother's group to make some friends in this city? I also worry that I'll have to work harder than ever at work, and at my friendships, to prove to everyone that nothing has changed because I'm now a mother. Will I bore my friends with talk of Baby Rowan? Why don't they ask about Baby Rowan? Is the nanny enjoying her job? Am I spending enough time with Baby Rowan? Is her head supposed to be that floppy? And I still don't know where the second, third, and fourth little piggies went and if that damn itsy-bitsy spider went up or down.

No, no, no. I'm not going to worry about how much more my life will change. I'm going to be a yummy mummy who has a fun career, fun friends, a great guy, and an adorable child who is well behaved, with a home in two cities.

I even send Cute Single Man an e-mail telling him that I'm coming to visit and that maybe we can go to a movie. Men will still be attracted to me, even if I'm a mother. Isn't fertility a turn-on? Perhaps, one day soon, I'll even get into that sexy dress I wore nine months ago at my engagement party, a.k.a. the Conception Party. (When am I going to find time to get married now?) It was a fabulous dress and should be seen. If I can find the dress. Though I wore it less than a year ago, it seems as though a lifetime has passed.

It's true that I no longer feel the need to go out and party every night. If I am away from Baby Rowan, even for a minute, I miss her. Coming home early, or not going out at all, won't be so bad knowing that Baby Rowan is home waiting for me.

But really, this baby is *not* going to change my life—well, not entirely. I'll still be *me*. You can quote me on that.

NOVEMBER 1

4:00 p.m.

"Hey, it's me," I say into the phone. I have called the fiancé at the office. I have a very important question that needs to be answered immediately.

"How's my baby?" he asks.

"Oh, I'm okay."

"No, I mean Rowan."

"Oh. She's fine." Is this how it's going to be from now on? "Listen, do you think that I look fat?"

"No, I don't. Beck, I have to work."

"Really, just tell me the truth. Do I look fat? You can tell me. Is my ass—Hello? Hello?"

ACKNOWLEDGMENTS

Thanks to Denise Bukowski, and the rest of the team at the Bukowski Agency, especially Jackie Joiner, for getting me motivated, forcing me to fill out the dreaded paperwork, and believing in me. To Maya Mavjee, Martha Kanya-Forstner, Stephanie Fysh, Scott Sellers, and the rest of the team at Doubleday, for being so nice and a pleasure to work with. Many thanks also to Allison Dickens. To the Girlfriends who make life easier and fun: Viia Beaumanis, Tassie Cameron, Liza Cooperman, Leanne Delap, Dara Fleischer, Sally Healy, Kim Izzo, Victoria Jackman, Louisa McCormack, Leah McLaren, Ceri Marsh, Jasmine Miller, Marcella Munro, Tralee Pearce, Sheri Segal, Tessa Sproule, Joanna Track, Kama

Truch, Dana Yanover-Fields, Tamar Zenith, and, especially, to my best friend and closest confidante, Rebecca Katz. To the Guyfriends: Allen Abel, Mark Gollom, Duncan Jackman, Mark Kingwell, Michael Martin, Andrew Pyper, Jacob Richler, Tim Rostron, Russell Smith, and, especially, to the real Cute Single Man for the Big Macs and watermelon. Thanks to the *National Post* and the Posties, notably Ben Errett and Sarah Murdoch. Many thanks also to the Ecklers: Lorne, Susan, Michael, Daniel, and Jon, and to my Zaida, Sam Burns, and to the Chetners, Glenda and Dave. Thanks to the mentors: Pamela Wallin, Dianne deFenoyl, Joan Crockatt, and Margaret Atwood. Many thanks to Dr. G. at Mount Sinai in Toronto and to Dr. B. at Foothills Hospital in Calgary. Big thanks to Imelda Acierda. And, of course, to the gym trainers: Sandra at Level V and Dawn at Heavens. My biggest and most heartfelt thanks for last: to Ken Whyte, to whom I owe absolutely everything. Thank you.

ABOUT THE AUTHOR

REBECCA ECKLER is a columnist with Canada's *National Post*, where she has been for four years, including a stint as a New York–based columnist and feature writer. She says she has the best job in the world. To read some of her recent articles, check out: www.nationalpost.com/commentary/reckler.html. Her work has also appeared in such publications as *Elle*, *Fashion*, *Lifestyles*, *Canadian House & Home*, and *Mademoiselle*. She moved to Calgary to be with her fiancé, who is the father of her baby daughter, Rowan. She is not planning on getting married anytime soon.